Ma Is Back!

Memoir of an Alzheimer's Discovery
Restoring My Mother's Memory

Brad Pitman   with Nancy A. Driscoll

ICAN, Ltd
Attleboro, MA USA

Copyright © 2010 by Bradford D. Pitman

Depend® is a registered trademark of Kimberly-Clark
Worldwide, Inc.

Published by:

ICAN, Ltd
Attleboro, Massachusetts
USA

Cover Art Concept and Design
Lisa Ramos

Cover Graphic Design
Kevin Ramos

Back Cover Design
Valerie Marak

Photo Credit
Kenneth Berman Photography

MAisBack.com

ISBN: 978-0-9830031-0-6

CONTENTS

DEDICATION

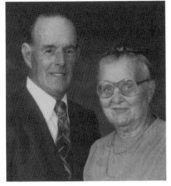

In the circle of life, there are few chances to honor those who created us. Seldom a time comes when we are prepared to meet the needs of our parents as they so readily met ours.

My mother, Maude Pitman's dementia gave me just such an opportunity. Without the formal and informal education she and my father, Bob Pitman, instilled in me, there would be no story.

Success was never assured, but without trying, failure was guaranteed. There was no choice but to try, and try we did. The result came without expectation, but turned out both surprising and pleasing.

I hope I have honored them.

Brad Pitman

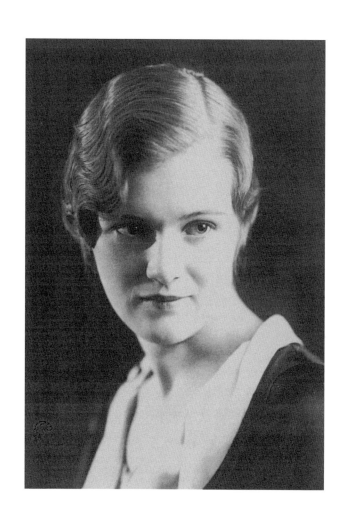

"Ma"

1931

Introduction

There was no easy or successful path to follow when I faced the reality that my mother, Maude Pitman, showed the first signs of senility, the term that was applied to the condition that affected certain elderly in the years long before I was born. My mother's senility became dementia and then, years later, we were faced with the frightening diagnosis of Alzheimer's Disease ("AD"). When first confronted with my mother's Alzheimer's, I viewed it as no different from my understanding of senility. The behavior was the same, and the treatment no more successful than in previous years. This presented a bleak outlook.

Every author, every professional, every friend and relative I encountered who had any connection to Alzheimer's Disease expressed a fatalistic acceptance of the diagnosis, and their only plan was to carry out a graceful demise. I was not willing to accept the professional community's outlook without making the effort to search for something, anything, that would help my mother, so I chose to set out on my own journey.

I remember the first time I climbed Mt. Washington in New Hampshire. I had been told about the view looking east, the sun coming up over the coast of New England, and the Atlantic Ocean stretching forever. I thought I would never get to the top, and when I finally arrived, the fog had settled in, obscuring everything. Disappointing, but I returned to enjoy that spectacle another time, and it was sweeter for my trouble.

The journey to help clear my mother's mind was shrouded in fog as well. There were stumbles and disappointments along the way, but once the peak was achieved, the view was far brighter for me than even that stunning New Hampshire vista.

SHOWERING

I heard the sound of my mother working her way down the hall outside my bedroom door. She appeared, steadying herself with the railing, and gave me a sly look that asked, "Is this the way to the bathroom?"

It was small acts like these that reminded me that my mother needed me as much as I had needed her when I was a child. Funny, how similar our needs are in the beginning of life and in old age, and nothing made that point clearer to me than showering Ma.

One would think it uncomfortable for a fifty-seven-year-old son to shower his mother, but the need was there and there was no question in my mind of how it was to be handled. It was a family trait to choose logic and reason over feelings of discomfort; there was a task that needed doing and, in my family, I was the guy who would get the job done.

Showering my mother fell into my hands quite naturally since I was the only one around to do it. My father had died nine years previously and my brother Bob, the oldest of my parents' three children, whose sickly childhood took much of my mother's time and attention, lived forty miles away, visiting only on weekends. My sister Kendra, the child who lit up my father with pride and perhaps vied with my mother for a place in his heart, lived over 100 miles away and was fully involved with children and grandchildren of her own.

I was the youngest of the three, and was told, "Brad, well, you were just there," by my sister, and I think accurately so. As far back as I can remember, I have no recollection of being put to bed, but do recall clearly doing the job myself, settling under the covers after several attempts to hoist myself into a bed that seemed mountainous to me. I also remember the first time I executed the leap easily, and the satisfaction I felt at accomplishing the feat. Do I suffer feelings of remorse, resentment, or neglect? I don't believe so. That was the way our household operated. I knew no other way, and accepted my place in the lineup.

Showering my mother was an impersonal event. While demented, she showed no signs of knowing who was helping her bathe or what was happening. At other times, when she was more alert, she would mimic my businesslike demeanor. We treated the situation as a simple necessity of circumstance.

I distinctly remember one day looking at her face while she was showering and seeing it with fresh vision. People would comment on my mother's smooth skin. I had known nothing else, but it did have a healthy look, especially for an eighty-four year old.

The face was the same, but who was this woman – my mother? There was no evidence at the moment of her former indomitable spirit. The woman who was at one time so obviously in charge now sat, expressionless, on the bath stool in the tub.

I shampooed her now sparse hair, and it took only a brief press of a towel to dry. The dent in her left temple was more evident now, the only aftereffect of the cerebral hemorrhage operation she had undergone eighteen years earlier. The doctor had said most people didn't live more than eight years after such an event, as they usually have another vascular problem that takes their lives. But here she was.

My mother's eyes were a soft blue, but lacked their characteristic liveliness. They once sparkled during the telling of a humorous story, or flashed when she made up her mind about something and was sticking to her guns no matter what the outcome. That spark had been replaced by vague staring or unknowing glances.

I washed her forearms and hands, familiar with the various-sized scars, trophies from her years of wrestling with rose bushes and branches. She had never pampered herself in the garden and a scratch or tear was left unattended until she was done. Her wrists were bony, the skin on her hands loose, paper-thin and translucent. Her rings had always remained on during whatever project or chore my mother did (taped over in the garden) and, as usual, they showered along with her, but were looser on her fingers now, turning easily with the action of the towel.

Ma's feet, size five, had always seemed small for her frame and her ankles were back, no longer bloated, but thin, perhaps her most delicate feature, except for her mind. During her shower she wasn't anxious or startled, and seemed happy to have me there guiding her. I was confident somehow that the trust she had always had in me was still present. All seemed familiar, I thought.

I washed her teeth in the morning and at night, and I did that now, recalling her past decision to choose the more expensive, natural-looking dentures when the time had

3

come. It was surprising to me because my mother had always been frugal and never fussed about appearances. I remembered that her attire was by choice always more practical than fashionable, dressing herself for the activity, be it gardening, boating, flying in my father's plane or for some social occasion. She was known to show up on the ski slope cloaked in an outdated mink coat, a camera strapped across her front, and what she referred to as her "snake bite kit," containing her lunch and various other essentials, around her waist. Less than typical for skiing, her attire served her purposes. But the teeth were another story, and my mother had gone ahead in her determined, self-assured way, and purchased the best dentures in the offing. These same dentures stayed in their tray now when not in use. After scrubbing them, I handed them to her, and she mechanically installed them herself, fumbling, dropping them, and finally wiggling them until they clicked into place. I thought of how many parts made one physically whole, but she was without her mind.

The final touch was brushing her hair. I fluffed it up and combed it into her usual style as best I could. Though sorely lacking in such skills, I clumsily did my best. It pleased me to make her look like herself, preserving what was there.

When the showering was done and Ma was groomed, I gave her a once-over and knew that in spite of the change in who was taking care of whom, regardless of the empty look in those blue eyes, and despite the uncharacteristic vulnerability of her pose, she was still my mother.

ADVENTURER

S omewhere deep inside this docile being, who silently endured her daily shower, was my mother, a former spitfire of a woman, intelligent, multi-talented, and an adventurer of sorts.

It is true that she stayed home, raised three children, and liked to sew, knit and garden. It is also true that, though it was sometimes not her direct choice, my mother did participate in more adventures than the average woman of her day.

As a young girl her family camped at Dolly Copp Campground near Mt. Washington in New Hampshire. Before she reached young adulthood, she had climbed every New England peak 4,000 feet and over with her father, two brothers and sister.

In her youth, my mother's family had lived on the road adjacent to my father's family in Attleboro, Massachusetts. She and my father knew each other, but became more familiar at an early age when my father, cocky and rambunctious, rode his bike through her perfect garden. He was stopped suddenly when she reacted by inserting a hoe through the spokes of his bicycle, bringing his intrusion to an abrupt stop. I suspect there was an immediate understanding that lasted right up until he died from cancer after 52 years of marriage.

Once she became Maude Pitman, she was in for a ride, and one that she didn't object to. Driving with my father was always a white-knuckled adventure, but she never said much despite the speed and imminent danger as he frequently careened along at 90 to over 100 miles per hour in the family car. He was in the habit of doing things at top speed, and she didn't seem to find this objectionable. My mother had learned to operate a car when she was thirteen and, in all her driving years, had gotten just one citation, a parking ticket. That one blemish on her record galled her for years, but my father's driving habits never got a rise out of her.

Dad was behind the wheel as usual on one of their spirited adventures. As they approached a bridge in New Hampshire on their way home from skiing, the car went into a spin. There was no use trying to stop the vehicle, so over the bridge they went, backwards. When they reached the other side, still on the roadway, my father gave the steering wheel a quick jerk, the car spun 180 degrees and they continued on their way. My mother sat in the passenger seat without comment. The reaction didn't seem to be from fright, but from confidence in the driver.

Cars didn't get my father where he wanted to go fast enough, so he bought a series of four planes during his lifetime, and my mother was on board during many of his excursions. Since these perilous trips were the norm in our family, we didn't recognize them as particularly hair-raising. Dad's seaplane was structured so that the hull landed on the water, with a pontoon on each wing for balance. Since my father's destinations often involved tight landings, occasionally in rough water, he managed to go through a total of nine pontoons, tearing them off one or two at a time, under a variety of difficult circumstances. My mother was with him for some of these flights, and was accustomed to my father running the plane lengthwise along four foot swells. Dad reported my mother's only comment during one such escapade, "There goes another pontoon, Robert!"

The plane had landing gear, wheels, which lowered for a terrain landing. Another time while attempting to land at the airport on Cape Cod, only one of the plane's wheels moved into place. He couldn't get the other one to release, nor would the first retract, making a water landing impossible and a ground landing problematic. His solution was to circle, make a landing approach, bump the ground with the single wheel, which snapped up into its recess as he had hoped, and then land the plane on its hull, on the ground, no wheels. This adventure didn't ruffle either of my parents and, I have a picture of my mother casually coiling up the sea plane's anchor line after they got it back onto its wheels. It was also not uncommon for my mother to be on board as he clickity-clacked through treetops coming out over the mountains surrounding the North Conway, New Hampshire airport.

Boating was a similar thrill. My mother liked to go to Nantucket on the weekends with my father in their 36-foot Sea Skiff. She was the pilot, and a very good one. During the first year of owning the boat, all of their ten or so trips to the island were made in near-zero visibility fog. This was viewed by my mother as an inconvenience, but certainly not a deterrent. Dad would be perched on the bow of the boat looking for buoys and listening for bells and fog horns, while she piloted by following the compass course he had set. Suddenly a buoy would be before them. "Reverse!" he would holler, and she would jam it into reverse.

The sound of the motor would often drown out his commands, so in order to avoid a disaster my father finally installed a communication device on the front of the boat. It was a trumpet-shaped horn that picked up the sound and transferred it to my mother. She could better hear his commands from the bow, and she could talk to him from the pilothouse. This type of navigation became commonplace for them, as not going due to fog wasn't a consideration. Once they made up their minds to go, they would be off!

It wasn't all madness while flying, boating or driving. There was always talk and adventures of the mind. Bob Allen, a longtime friend and participant in the family fun, still tells stories about my parents and their freewheeling way of life. He reminisces about ski trips to New Hampshire in the family car where my father would do the driving, and Bob and my mother would do the talking. He loved her stories and jokes, and appreciated her willingness to listen to his.

One of Bob's favorite stories shows an appreciation for my mother's analytical mind. In the car on the way up north, he had posed a question. "There are only two places in the world where the American flag is flown day and night. Can you name them?" As he tells it she, of course, came up with the White House right away, but continued to mull the problem over, even after a few later runs down the mountain. She finally got the answer – over the grave of Francis Scott Key. Bob likes to say that he has asked that question frequently, but claims my mother was the only one to get it right. It is one of the many stories Bob tells as an example of how my mother's sharp mind elevated mere travel to an adventure.

He also fondly recounts when my mother, father, he, and others formed the Attleboro Ski Club in 1948. In the early stages they met at the Attleboro YMCA and, then, when their numbers grew, they moved to the Attleboro Grange Hall, where they planned ski trips and socialized. Later when my parents were in their seventies and my mother's skiing days were behind her, the ski club members made my father and her honorary members, and she continued to visit and enjoy the camaraderie and exchange of past ski adventures.

An old note from my mother to my father illustrates her ever-ready spirit of adventure. I came across the yellowing piece of loose-leaf paper while purging a room of clutter. I don't know when it was written, but knowing Ma, it could have been almost any day of any week of her life with my father. Written in red marker, an extra-large version of my mother's clear script filled the page.

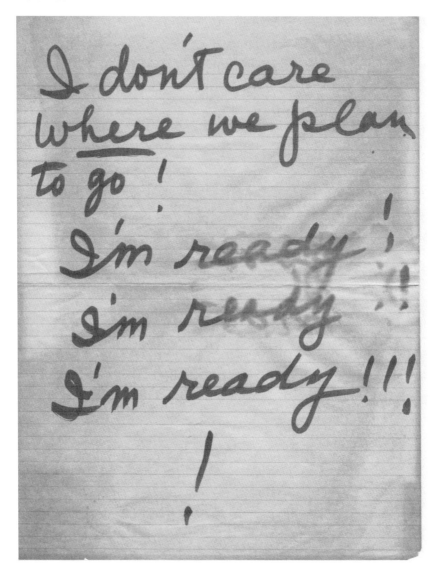

She had always been ready. But this silent, spirit-less woman who allowed me to tend to her in 1996 seemed but a faded shadow of the mother whose vitality and vivaciousness was but a persistent memory.

BACK HOME AGAIN

I had not always lived with my mother. I divorced after ten years of marriage, prior to my mother's diagnosis of Alzheimer's Disease. It was with great regret that I left the household of my seven-year old daughter Annie, but circumstances were such that it happened that way. Since then I had lived in two different houses, one I had built on five acres of land. In two years I had the gardens looking like those I grew up with and, though I enjoyed the yard work, I was also taking care of my mother's yard, as well as her beach house, and making my living developing land and selling real estate.

In 1991 my mother and I agreed that it made sense for me to move into her house, my childhood home in Attleboro, Massachusetts. At this point she had not shown any obvious signs of dementia, but her 79 years were beginning to take their toll, and a congestive heart condition was changing her life. Maintaining three households had become unreasonable. I had no idea what her financial situation was and she was not about to discuss it. I had reason to question this as she had also been talking about selling the house on Cape Cod, and I thought I might help delay that. And so, at age 52, I took up residency in my old room, a move I hadn't exactly envisioned for myself, but one that I made without regret. Did I move in for the express purpose of caring for her? No. But I was aware of the probability that I would be needed in the not-too-distant future.

A TYPICAL DAY

It was not my way to become emotional about the situation, or spend time mourning the loss of who my mother had been. It was, and still is, not in my makeup, and I showed my emotion and caring by doing the job at hand.

I have a dreamlike, nightmarish recollection of what life was like in our household when my mother was at her worst, approximately one year after her Alzheimer's diagnosis in 1996. Though this is her story, I was her caregiver. So her story is also mine. Looking back, I don't know how I functioned; but, as many who care for their elderly loved ones do, I put one foot in front of the other, and didn't spend much time fretting about the situation.

Though the sun rose and set, there was no morning, no night, no start, no finish, just endless time and tasks. Breakfast, lunch and supper came in a continuous cycle between snatched rest: five minutes here, fifteen minutes there or, if I was lucky, maybe an hour of precious uninterrupted sleep.

I kept the routine of an early breakfast. The sun was up and so was I, and at this time my mother might be more alert than not, as it was her best time of day.

The pre-breakfast routine would begin. Get her untangled from the sheets and unknot the nightie. Time to change her and get her ready to go downstairs. It was off to the bathroom where she needed to be washed. Some days it was as little as washing her face; others it was into the tub for the full treatment.

I put on her clothes, layer upon layer, Depends, undergarments, shirt. She would be dressed enough to be warm while I worked on putting on those compression socks. No, she wanted her robe first. So, the robe it was. The stockings, which were to keep the fluid in her legs from settling and causing her ankles and calves to swell, were the real challenge as at first the doctor had prescribed the tightest strength, the most difficult to put on. I would often spend fifteen or twenty minutes struggling with them, but they proved to be impossible as they hurt her and frustrated me. The less taut variety became the only ones I could use. As I wrestled with the hose, every crease or wrinkle in them had to be smoothed or they would hurt her and cut off her circulation.

In my mind I could imagine my mother in her better days saying something like "Why are you 'wrastling' with those socks?", but there were no feigned dialects or funny expressions coming from her at this time. Socks on, then pants, sweater and, finally, her shoes.

I took inventory – teeth, hearing aids, glasses, and then the things that beautify – hair combed, nails cleaned, cut and filed smooth. Toenail care was slid in any time I could get away with doing it. I marveled at the parts it took to put her back together, all the while thinking that when I got older I'd become more of a construction job as well. Nothing brings you face-to-face with your own mortality like participating in the daily piece-by-piece reassembly of a parent.

The trip down to breakfast was no easy task. The stairs in our house have two left turns on wedge-shaped stairs, with the handrail on the narrow inside. They were treacherous even under the best of circumstances. I had a rail installed on the wall at the wide side of the stairs, so I could now guide her down them more safely.

With my mother sitting at the kitchen table, it was time for her breakfast. It was easy to feed her breakfast, as she ate the same thing, day after day, week after week, year after year, and I didn't change the routine. Though her breakfast food didn't fit into part of my theory of feeding her just the "good" stuff, it worked. Two cups of decaffeinated coffee and her favorite raspberry danish. She loved it, so she got it. As she ate, so did I.

She got pineapple juice with her pills. I didn't bother trying to understand why she chose to take her pills by lining them up and lapping them up right off the table. It wasn't pretty, and the old Ma would have been horrified to see herself, but it worked, the chore of getting the pills into her was achieved, and I wasn't about to fight success. I justified letting this happen with the recollection of her former adage that a few germs wouldn't kill you and might even give you some natural immunity, and I was just plain tired.

It was soon time for another change and cleanup, maybe even before she finished breakfast. She got fresh Depends and sometimes clean slacks, and maybe a new set of pressure stockings if the occasion called for it. Clothes and bed linens piled up quickly and the chug and whirr of the washer and dryer was a constant background sound in the house. A quick tidying of the bathroom and it was ready for her next visit.

We continued down the back hall into the living room where my mother took her customary seat on the couch in front of the television. Nothing had been moved, so everything was familiar, but I knew she really had no idea where she was, or even that she owned the house. It was all just beyond her. I turned on the TV, even though she didn't know it existed, because it fulfilled my need to stimulate all of her senses: sound, in this case.

Our dog, Ooste, had to be fed and taken out to do her business. It was fitted in when I could, or as needed.

A knock on the door announced the visiting nurse's brief call. I paused my routine and welcomed her to do her work: draw blood to be tested to determine Coumadin levels, check my mother's legs for swelling, and take her vitals. This occurred once or twice a week, and small signs from my mother made me believe she was comfortable with these interactions.

My own work would call again, as it was approaching winter and I had to coordinate making the ski equipment I manufacture. I would die-cut the material, get the parts to the sewers, retrieve the finished product, fold, pack, take the orders and ship them. The job wasn't performed with any continuity as my mother needed her tonic water with lemonade, and then another Depends change, sometimes immediately. I had to keep her dry or the ever-threatening urinary tract infection might return. I would tend to her, and then resume my work.

At times my ski business ran simultaneously with real estate sales and land development. To the extent time allowed, I bought, subdivided, and sold a few small parcels during my mother's health problems. But it wasn't quite that simple. One parcel required getting wetlands approval before I could clean up the dead trees and brush. I fit these business tasks in wherever I could. At first I did all there was to be done with my mother's care as I had to have an understanding of what worked. With my mother's care being first priority, it eventually became obvious I would need help. I hired a caregiver, Cheryl Neal, who had prior experience as a nursing home aide. She was kind and attentive, and was just what my mother needed. Cheryl would arrive at 9 a.m. and take my place so I could tend to my business. Though still pressured, I could now create ads, show property, write sales agreements and transfer titles while Cheryl was there for my mother.

Then there were the gardens, the ones my mother had spent forty or more hours a week in during spring, summer and fall. Daytime was often too short, so I worked them by floodlight, early morning or in the evening, but daylight was needed to mow the grass and trim the edges. No weeds were allowed, and being true to the other part of my theory, keeping the "bad" out of my mother's life, no chemicals were used. Weeding was done by hand. The grass was so lush weeds didn't have much of a chance, but less so when I saw them. Then there were the shrubs that were 50 years old and wanted tender loving care. Those days were busy, but the gardens and yard were relaxing and beautiful, and they supplied the house with the flowers my mother had loved and nurtured for so many years – another comfortable, familiar part of her life.

Cheryl went home at about two or three in the afternoon; afterward, I was back full time with my mother. I did more laundry and changed the beds, and her.

Between changes, she sat slumped on the couch in a stupor.

Next on the agenda was the evening meal. It almost always included fresh vegetables with fish or chicken, and occasionally red meat. Yellow corn on the cob showed up two or three times per week, winter, spring, summer or fall. Spaghetti sauce took time to prepare, so I made large quantities and froze it to be used later in meatloaf, on chicken or pasta.

I knew a microwave would be easier, but I chose not to have one.

I would wake my mother up, get her to the table, and serve dinner. Though I tried, there was no conversation or interaction at this point, and this quiet followed us into the living room where she would sit in an Alzheimer's daze until bedtime.

Then there was night. I would get my mother upstairs, washed, changed, and to bed with clean Depends, nightie on, the rubber pad under the sheet, and chucks, the disposable waterproof pads, on top. On a bad night, it was on to chasing the demons in her head, as she hallucinated about frightening, crawly things. Her yelling was distracting, always disturbing, and part of my very worst nights. All I could do was listen and try to calm her. She would be in bed for fifteen minutes and then up again. Sometimes it seemed she was on a trampoline as she no sooner hit the sheets than she was up and walking. It was seldom that she would remain in bed for a straight two hours.

All night it was in and out of bed, to change her, sometimes change the bed, and straighten it out so she wasn't trapped in the sheets or blankets. Breakfast time arrived before I knew it, so day and night became one long event of changing, feeding, cleaning, and stealing a few minutes of rest.

In my "spare time" I read the newspaper, food shopped, paid the bills, did bookkeeping for my mother and me, and attended to any other little things that came up.

Though this may sound like a litany of complaint, it is not. What I was doing was what a mother, or anyone else who cares for a family while holding down a job, does. I did not consider it a burden; it was just life. Again, it was in keeping with our family dynamic that this should be my role, and one that I stepped into without a second thought.

WHO'S THAT?

My brother Bob came down on Friday nights to spend weekends with our mother. His time here gave me a little relief and a chance to work in the yard and clean the house. His visits also provided me with a break from the stress of constantly attempting to improve the situation.

A trip to the local pancake house for dinner would kick off their weekend. This was a continuation of my parents' and Bob's previous habit, which he kept up even after my father's death in 1987. Bob thought it was a good idea to keep the tradition and so did I.

Interestingly enough, before Alzheimer's changed her life, she was walking poorly. My mother would totter out to the driveway with assistance on her Friday night trek to supper with Bob and, when she encountered any ants on the pavement, she would persist in her longtime habit of squashing each and every one of them. For whatever reason, my mother carried on a lifelong vendetta against ants. Though a danger to herself because she no longer had the coordination for the activity, she would dance about, swaying and stomping her feet emphatically down upon the scurrying victims. In order to prevent a catastrophe, we were careful to be at hand. After annihilating the ants, she would shuffle the rest of the way to the car.

I often thought about how surprising it was that the body sometimes follows the motivation of the mind, and my mother's desire to rid the world of ants seemed to give her the energy and ability to move quickly and with a gusto that was missing from her everyday gait.

At the restaurant my mother ordered her usual Friday night favorite, waffles with strawberries and whipped cream. I could always tell what she had to eat, as she wore it well.

Many weekends Bob would take her for a ride to see the sights that were familiar to her. The season would dictate the tour: gardens, snowy sights, cemeteries, or our old house by the sea. Stimulation of this kind was enjoyed by both of them.

However, these visits came with a price. Bob, like the rest of the family, didn't know when to stop talking. During his weekend visits he would talk about all sorts of things and, as Alzheimer's advanced, my mother would sit there with little reaction or offer disconnected responses. He did not seem to fully comprehend that my mother did not really know who he was, or that she was as bad off as she was.

Sometimes while watching game shows on television, he would argue with her when she made no sense, failing to understand that arguing with someone in her condition was futile. The worst part was he did not see that this type of interaction made her anxious and upset. No matter what I tried, I was unable to stop these exchanges.

One Sunday, Bob arose to go home around noontime after what had proved to be a trying weekend. After he exited, Ma turned to me and asked, "Who is that chatty little man?"

My immediate thought was, "I wonder what she would say about me when I leave?" This struck me as tragically funny. I hung on to the humor so as not to be overcome with sadness and a sense of futility.

Bob was her first child and so few words told so much about where my mother was at that point in time. She did not know him or me, nor did she recognize the house she was sitting in.

During this period it seemed that my brother's good intentions and the break in her routine exhausted my mother. She would be spent on Mondays, arising later than usual, and she would have more difficulty in doing what she had done easily the Friday before. Tuesday's improvement featured her sleeping less than Monday, and her walking around the house would increase. By Wednesday she would be back to her previous state; Thursday and Friday brought improvements, and then the cycle would begin again.

Down the road, as my mother made positive strides with her dementia, there appeared to be no tiring effects from these weekend visits.

THE WORST OF TIMES

P eople who are caring for loved ones plummeting in a downward Alzheimer's spiral often hit a pivotal point where they feel overwhelmed by the condition and the chaos that accompanies it. We hit just such a low point in dealing with my mother's disease, and it felt like rock bottom.

I had been living with my mother for five years; she was 84, I was 57, and we had been going along with the ups and downs connected with Alzheimer's Disease for several months. It seemed to me that the conventional wisdom was to accept the mental lapses that accompanied the disease but to ignore the bright flashes of mental acuity that also happened. These isolated moments were dismissed by our medical contacts as flukes, or simply evidence of imbedded long-term memory. I had been encouraged by some bright moments in my mother's days. These flashes of sharp-mindedness occurred without medication, and I felt that they came from the genius of the human body and its resilient ability to use all that was within to attempt a correction of ill health. To build on this I had developed a theory that concentrated on the moments of wellness, rather than the lapses. I felt that there must be a reason for such lucid moments, and I had done much research and made adjustments in her diet and lifestyle as a result. The details of these adjustments follow later in this book.

However, on the day our lives unraveled completely, her colitis and incontinence were raging, and she needed to be changed a dozen times. That night was just as bad, and she and her sheets had required changing three more times. Though she usually needed help walking, my mother had been in and out of bed. I found her standing next to her bed a few times, and I helped her back in. She was having hallucinations about insects on the ceiling; she screamed and yelled, pointing here and there, as she directed me to swat or kill the bugs. Though I looked in the direction indicated, for the most part, I didn't react. It was impossible not to be upset by the frantic, hysterical emotions she displayed, but I subdued my feelings, knowing there was no benefit to becoming sidetracked with emotions of my own.

I was exhausted and, during a moment of reprieve, I dozed off for a few minutes. I awakened to find her holding onto the bathroom doorjamb. How she managed to get herself into the bathroom was beyond my understanding.

It reminded me that though it was only months before that she had been visiting the bathroom unassisted, there was one night when she had gotten into the bathroom, was unable to get out, and had entangled her feet in the rug. I rescued her, removed the rug, and that was that.

Now, as she stood in that same doorway, her brain seemed unable to tell her feet to move. I asked, I begged her to try to move, and struggled to come up with a way to get her back to her bedroom. I couldn't lift or carry her, nor did I have a wheelchair. I tried everything I could to maneuver her toward her room. I attempted to move her legs with my hands. I tried bending her legs by gently nudging then from behind while holding her to keep her from falling. She was absolutely rigid, as immoveable as a stone statue. I was exhausted, bewildered, and almost defeated.

Using every method I could think of, I inched her into the hallway, maneuvering her past the open stairway where I feared a headlong fall if either of us weakened. The distance from bathroom to bedroom of some 20 feet took an hour and forty-five minutes.

Once we got into the bedroom, instead of making it to the bed, she dropped down into a chair. It was 4:20 in the morning, and since I hadn't slept much, I was unable to help her achieve the last leg of the journey from chair to bed. The commotion we had made roused my brother Bob, who was there for his usual weekend visit. He came into the room and tried to help.

In the midst of our attempts to get her to the bed, my mother became aggressive and attacked him. My brother was holding her right arm as we steered her toward the bed. With her mouth open and teeth bared, she suddenly made an aggressive head-bob in his direction, attempting to sink her teeth into his forearm.

Bob was obviously shaken by the attack, and forgetting that this was his mother, screamed, "I'll break your f***ing arm!"

The chaos of the scene suddenly came into full focus for me. Not only was my mother unmanageable, but my brother was out of control as well, and I again felt overwhelmed with the fear of having to deal with the situation for even one more day. We had tumbled into the bleakest of life's low points, and I had had enough. I decided that my mother was going to the hospital.

HOSPITALIZATION

That same day, my mother was checked into the hospital, where she would remain for a total of twelve days. She had been assigned Dr. Sullivan as her primary care physician. He immediately recognized the serious problem of her poorly treated congestive heart failure, and dealt with it by using Lasix, to take off excess fluid. We had to be careful of the electrolytes and blood chemistry, as her potassium could drop to levels that would have ended everything. The doctor added potassium in a form we could mix with her daily liquids at home.

Dr. Sullivan reinforced my understanding of the importance of drinking sufficient liquids to avoid the danger of dehydration that Lasix could precipitate. In addition, he added folic acid, vitamin C, and baby aspirin to her daily intake of medications and supplements.

While in the hospital she shed more than 16 pounds of fluid, and her heart medication was adjusted. As soon as Ma lost this fluid, her hallucinations lessened. It was obvious that her care for this problem had previously been ineffective, and I had also been concerned that her load of heart medication could have been part of her memory problem. At this point I was convinced that, had Dr. Sullivan not taken these steps, our battle would have had a much steeper uphill slope.

Dr. Sullivan had worked his magic with my mother's condition and she was as medically sound as she possibly could be, though her dementia persisted. She was not exactly healthy, but all we could do was pay attention and make sure she did not succumb to further urinary tract infections, dehydration, and electrolyte imbalances.

She was moved to a neuro-psych geriatric ward for Alzheimer's care, and I went in to see her mid-afternoon to find her confined to a wheelchair – but there was another problem as well. There was another patient, a woman, in front of my mother, staring at her. The lady obviously had mental issues; her hair was a wild wiry field of grey, her moist eyes were unfocused, and she was nose-to-nose with Ma. I could see that my mother was frightened, a state so uncharacteristic of this once-fearless woman. I immediately moved the wheelchair away from the woman. She followed us, attempting to keep up the face-to-face contact with my mother. She was talking and gesturing erratically and following our every move.

After what seemed longer than it actually was, an attendant came to our rescue.

My mother looked up at me, and in a clear, lucid voice asked, "What have I done to deserve this? Get me out of here."

I was caught off guard by the sheer heartbreak the scene produced in me, and was unable to respond.

Though I knew I would bring my mother home, I had to make plans for her sudden unexpected return. I told her I just could not do it right then, but I would be back at nine the next morning to get her. I informed the attendant, and he said they couldn't have her ready by then.

"I'll get her ready myself if you haven't done it by that time," I said.

I was told that I would be unable to take care of her at home.

"I've been told that before."

First the nurses attempted to dissuade me, then the social worker, and, when the doctor wasn't available, they said they would have him call me.

"I'll be here at nine. Have her ready." I left.

In my eyes the ward was chaotic, the exact opposite of the calm, familiar environment that I believed was best for my mother.

I arrived at nine the following morning to find that she had not been dressed. The nurse said the doctor wanted to talk to me. I told her that he could talk to me while I got my mother ready and, if they weren't agreeable to that, I would leave with her, as is. They quickly began to attend to her.

The doctor came along and continued the lecture begun by other hospital staff, and the aides slowed down in getting my mother ready. I was not in agreement and got up in the middle of the talk. Everyone then understood that the game was up and we were leaving. They got her ready immediately, and we exited.

It is true that we had reached a crucial place on that dreadful night twelve days before, but with my spirit recharged and my resolve renewed, we set out for home and a new course of treatment.

Simultaneous with our escape from the neuro-psych ward, we had to address a problem with Risperdal, the drug that had been used to control my mother's hallucinations. The neurologist had prescribed one milligram, but this amount knocked her out. After consulting with Dr. Sullivan and the pharmacist, we adjusted her Risperdal to one half of a milligram. She appeared less zonked, so after a trip back to the doctor and pharmacist, we lowered the dose to one quarter of a milligram. The medication only came in one mg tablets, so this involved quartering the tablet. The measurement was not very exact, but it soon made no difference because when her congestive heart failure was better controlled, and the urinary tract infections held at bay, she was calm. After a short time, we stopped the Risperdal altogether. My mother never had another hallucination.

Gardens

W hen I brought my mother home from the hospital, it was autumn. The chrysanthemums were fading away and as I covered them before winter hit, as always, I thought of my mother and her gardens.

A garden was always in her and thus a constant in my life as well. The garden where she and my father had their first meeting of wills was her first. She was about nine or ten, and it was in that garden that she first bred some roses, and raised a variety of blossoms that surrounded her rows of vegetables. Later in life, when an old friend casually mentioned it in conversation, the topic of her cross-breeding of a few types of roses in her youth, she quickly dismissed it. She wasn't one to dwell on her accomplishments, and didn't expect others to either. From this young age, a garden was her comfort zone. When I came along, since she spent most of the daylight caring for her plants, I was brought up in the garden.

In 1943 during the Second World War, my mother had a Victory garden in a vacant lot across the street from our house and it was the setting of some of my earliest memories. She raised string beans, onions, carrots, potatoes, peas, beets, and a single turnip (for my father), along with some flowers.

My brother and sister were in school during the day, so, in my preschool years, the garden was my playground and, in a different way, I suppose, my mother's as well.

She had a hose that she dragged from the spigot on our house across the street to her Victory garden, and my parents had fashioned a wooden trough of sorts under which they ran the hose. The trough was, of course, to protect the hose when cars came down the street. I can still recall my attempts and my inability to pull the hose and the wooden covering across the road, "helping" my mother. I watered the plants at times, getting unrecognizably muddy, something that didn't bother her in the least. Other times I would plant myself on the dirt sidewalk, digging holes and making mounds, imagining highly developed constructions in my handiwork. Occasionally I was given a few pea seeds or some potato sprouts to plant. She was no doubt trying to entertain me and simultaneously indoctrinate me into proper gardening.

Other times I was chastised, once for trampling hyacinths and tulips in my bungling attempts to participate, another time for cutting a perfectly good potato in half in my enthusiasm to unearth them with a hoe. My mother was frugal, and we made sure we ate that one immediately.

The first flowers she taught me to plant were pansies. She told me they were the first flower her grandmother always put in, as did her mother, and so did she. I feel satisfaction in perpetuating the tradition, and I have noticed that my daughter has begun planting pansies in the spring with her two girls.

Later, after I had outgrown tagging along in the garden, she established a garden at our Cape house. I call it the Cape house, but it was really nothing more than a cabin – our summer headquarters nonetheless. My mother liked it because it was "rustic," meaning she could simply take a broom and sweep the sand right out the door. Her garden was about 150 feet from the cabin, up the dirt drive, around the gazebo, the bay inlet on its left. She spent hours in this garden as well, raising her usual assortment of vegetables and many rather frustratingly unsuccessful attempts at corn. She blanched and stored these vegetables in the freezer in the basement. She also grew flowers around the gazebo and the cabin, and oftentimes would wander back from boat trips with my father directly into the gardens to weed and water. The care of the vegetables and flowers was not a chore, but a pleasure for my mother.

She became well known for her flowers at home in Attleboro, and people would come from distances to view her roses and especially her iris gardens.

After my mother's death, Cheryl, her caregiver and friend, told me about some of their conversations of which I was unaware. When my mother's mental state had improved and she grew alert, she would reminisce about her membership in the Iris Club, commonly ending these anecdotes with a comment like, "You'd meet some real characters in that place!" When Ma made such remarks to me, I'd suggest that club members might be thinking the same in her regard.

Of course, by the time Cheryl came into the picture, I had taken over the care of the gardens. After my mother's health improved and I could devote more time to them, they were looking pretty darned good. In spite of my consistent ministering, though, my mother and I both knew that they were slightly shy of her meticulous standards. She was very kind about the difference, and there was a silent understanding between us concerning her appreciation for the care I took with them, and an acceptance that, though not quite up to her high mark, the gardens were just fine.

One day during Cheryl's shift, my mother decided she wanted to go outside and survey things, and expressed this wish to Cheryl, who agreed. Ma foraged around in her piles of gardening information and came up with her sketch of the layout, a very detailed diagram of the plots, with everything meticulously labeled.

She scavenged further and, true to her penchant for dressing for the occasion, she produced two rather unattractive sun hats, plopped one on her head, and insisted Cheryl wear the other. By then Cheryl knew better than to resist the will of Maude, so she put it on. It had a plastic seagull on the top of it, with some plastic sea horses and shells on the brim.

Once in the garden Ma systematically reviewed each of the many plants. She examined the individual nameplates that she had inserted into the ground years before, and seemed satisfied that everything was in order. Years later, Cheryl confided that, much to her embar-rassment, when I returned home from work, they were still in the yard wearing their unfashionable hats. I hadn't noticed.

And so, for almost her entire lifetime, except for the months when she was absent from us and from herself, my mother was content to devote hours among her flowers and vegetables. Without her garden, she was not complete.

Signs

Though my mother's mental acuity problems weren't apparent until approximately two years after I moved back into the old homestead, as I look back now, I might have had reason to suspect that she had a problem developing well before she was diagnosed.

One day, I entered the house and she was sitting at the kitchen table with a fish-shaped cutting board I had made her in the fourth grade. She had a hammer and nail and was pounding holes through some tags she was using in the garden. She was splitting the tail of the fish in the process! I tried, but could not stop her. I recognized that this was not the action of a woman who never threw away a functional object, nor would she mindlessly destroy one, particularly a hand-made gift from her son. I thought her actions were odd, and left, feeling hurt and confused.

Another day in 1995 I arrived home from work to find my mother face up in the garden.

"What are you doing on those iris?" I called, somewhat indelicately.

"Get me out of here. Now!" she demanded, explaining that some character had walked right by and didn't even stop to assist her.

As it turned out, her heart had been stopping, and in November of 1995 a pacemaker was installed. During the five months that followed, I observed more obvious signs of a problem with her thinking and behavior, but I suspected that the anesthesia administered during the pacemaker procedure might have contributed to the problem, as I thought this was always a possibility, especially in the elderly.

About the same time the pacemaker was installed, my mother was diagnosed with macular degeneration, which leads to gradual and progressive loss of sight. Later, after her Alzheimer's Disease diagnosis, I noted at AD meetings that several people I encountered who had been diagnosed with Alzheimer's also had age-related macular degeneration. No surprise there, as they were elderly. However, I also learned that these macular degeneration patients were previously taking a daily vitamin with 100% of the recommended daily allowance of zinc, and after their macular degeneration diagnosis, they were given a supplement with another large amount of zinc. Was there a connection between high doses of zinc and dementia? I didn't know but later, as her behavior changed, I considered everything suspect as a possible cause, so I found a one-a-day vitamin without zinc.

There were other small aberrations of behavior which wouldn't seem unusual to anyone who didn't know my mother well. I would find a tool she'd left in the garden, the water would still be on in the yard when I returned from work, or kitchen utensils would be in different places. I noticed these things, and chose to overlook them, thinking she must have had reasons for her uncharacteristic actions.

Were these the first signs she was becoming someone other than the person she had always been? I now suspect so. At that time I had no understanding of the significance or the consequences of this behavior. Even if I had, it would not have changed the course of our story.

As time went on, however, I began to suspect my mother was having trouble. In spite of the opinions of friends and relatives that nothing was wrong, I knew something was amiss. I simply failed to recognize where this out-of-character behavior was pointing.

Over the next year I became more and more convinced that my mother had a significant memory problem. I noticed a change in her ability to do her personal bookkeeping. Previously she would balance her books without ever using an adding machine or calculator; her work was flawless, and done with ease. Now her bookkeeping often sat on the kitchen table, unfinished, for a week, sometimes longer. The impact of this reminded me that she had been doing bookkeeping with efficiency since her marriage in 1935. She had frequently mentioned this fact and, in addition, I had discovered her old records stored in the attic. This was the same person who had skipped high school, graduated from Bryant & Stratton Business School (now Bryant University), at age 15 and later from Rhode Island School of Design at age 19. She had never had a problem with bookkeeping. Never! Something wasn't right.

During this same time period, prior to her initial diagnosis, I also noticed she had developed trouble recalling the names of people she knew. My mother was always brilliant at remembering names.

There was one time in the late forties when she was sitting in the car with us kids waiting for my father. It was a cold winter day, and we were parked on a dirt road on some land that my father was interested in buying. Dad had walked a ways into the woods to talk to the owner, who was cutting wood, and had unthinkingly taken the keys with him. He wasn't gone long before we all started shivering. We had no heat, and my mother was none too happy. When the two men finally approached the car, my father said "Maude, I want you to meet…"

"We're freezing. Give me the key. We want heat."

"Harold Brown," my father finished.

"Hi," was the only word my mother offered Mr. Brown, and it was their single meeting.

Thirty years later, when Dad was talking about the land off Hurricane Mountain Road in North Conway, New Hampshire he asked, "Maude, what was that guy's name?"

"How do I know? Oh, it was Harold Brown." She was able to toss the name out three decades later after only the briefest encounter.

Now, her inability to come up with a familiar name was out of the ordinary for her, and I couldn't help but notice her loss of that capacity.

My mother's problems had beginnings, I soon realized. Long before she lost her mental acuity, she lost her sense of smell. In 1994, before her diagnosis of Alzheimer's, it became apparent to me that something was odd when our dog Ooste's hair-curling, tail-end emissions produced absolutely no reaction from my mother. While anyone else in the room would dart to a window to let fresh air in after such explosions, her olfactory recognition was nil.

Though such an event might normally be accepted without worry, my thinking was that she had lost one of her senses and, since it is a function of the brain, I wanted it checked out. Though loss of sense of smell is now sometimes associated with Alzheimer's Disease, at the time I don't believe the connection had been made. Also my mother had previously suffered a cerebral hemorrhage and a stroke, and I was concerned about whether her loss of smell indicated a new brain problem. We took her to Massachusetts General Hospital to see a neurologist and a brain scan was done. The result was they saw no problem.

We continued with life as usual and, though she appeared well, my suspicions of a looming problem would soon be confirmed.

Role Changes

For a couple of years prior to there being any question as to my mother's competence, she had planned to sell the Cape house that my grandfather built in the 1920's. When I moved back into the family home, I had the notion that I may be able to relieve any financial pinch she might be having, and perhaps forestall its sale. My mother's mind was made up though – she was selling. Two years before, she had been very specific in her wishes and had told me the exact selling price she wanted and that she would not settle for less.

Because I had concerns about my mother's encroaching dementia, I wanted to meet with her attorney. He hesitated to meet, as he could not conceive that she was any less cogent than she had been just a few months before. He had been her lawyer for thirty years, and whenever she entered his office, she would comment, "How much is this going to cost me?" Their last encounter had been typical of years of good-natured give and take.

I insisted they meet, mentioning to him that she was having unusual problems with her bookkeeping. That didn't carry much weight. I told him I was still concerned that there was a problem as her doctor had indicated she knew my mother was having trouble understanding her pill schedule. This didn't impress him either. We visited him at his office and they bantered back and forth. She didn't miss a beat. He could see nothing wrong with her competence, as my mother was having one of her good days. There was no appearance of her having any mental malfunction, but I knew there were more problems than he perceived.

I was still concerned about future questions of competence, but I was armed with her attorney's opinion, and the authority was already in place for me to act on her behalf. It was unnecessary for me to go through the legal steps to secure power of attorney because years before when I gave my parents a trip to Europe, their wills were written, powers of attorney were established, and last medical wishes stipulated.

I went ahead with the plan to sell the house on the Cape, and found a buyer for it at the price my mother wanted. She attended the closing, made sure the selling price was correct, signed the deed, and closed the sale.

The sale of the summer house would prove to be the last important thing she did before her good judgment disappeared entirely.

TENTATIVE DIAGNOSIS

M uch had transpired in the years prior to my mother's infirm state in 1996. In 1988, three years before I moved back into her home, my mother's local doctor had been unable to address her mobility issues. We needed to get to the cause of why she was unable to take more than one step up at a time and, partly because of what seemed like my mother's unrealistic stubbornness, we needed to get to the cause in a timely manner.

I entered the house for a visit one day and my mother, who was 76 years old at the time, was sitting at the kitchen table surrounded by pamphlets touting European ski trips. I asked her what she was doing.

"I'm going to Austria and Italy."

"Ma, you can't even climb two stairs at a time." I responded.

"I don't care. I'm going and your brother is going with me."

"What good is that? He can hardly take care of himself!"

"I'm going."

She had gone to Austria and Switzerland in 1968 and she now was determined to go back with the same group of people she and my father had traveled with years before.

"Well, then I'll go along and take care of both of you," I said. My daughter, Anne, and I suddenly had a ski trip ahead of us.

In anticipation of the trip, we set out to find some way for my mother to improve her walking. We went to Massachusetts General Hospital ("MGH") and ended up with Dr. Carol Ehrlich, an internist who also taught at Harvard Medical School. She examined my mother thoroughly and immediately adjusted her medications.

Two months later, my mother was walking up stairs fairly well and getting around much better, though she would have gone to Europe even if she hadn't had this improvement. I learned much later that, before my father's death, my parents had made plans to revisit the area, and it seemed that my mother's determination to carry out their intentions had something to do with honoring him in her own way. We all went on the trip, had a great time, and my mother walked up and down the streets of Kitzbuhel, Austria, and St. Ulrich, Italy.

This was how our relationship with Dr. Ehrlich began. She was the right person at the right time, and so, when, about eight years later, signs were pointing that my mother was having memory problems, Dr. Ehrlich was still her doctor.

In early 1995, four years after I had returned to my mother's home, I began noticing that she was having trouble understanding her prescription medicine regime. She was sometimes confused about when to take this, or why she was taking that. Uncharacteristically, she had to consult her written medication schedule in the filling of her Sunday through Saturday pill organizer, and was even having some trouble while using the list. I noted this, but others, not privy to such daily habits, saw nothing wrong with her wit or behavior.

Dr. Ehrlich had been observing this type of behavior in my mother and started hinting that we may be seeing a dementia problem.

I took my mother to some preliminary testing for memory problems, but it didn't sink in until the day Dr. Ehrlich informed me, "Your mother has probable Alzheimer's." Of course I had heard of it, but I asked for a clear explanation of the disease and what it would mean for us.

"Your mother may know you today, but tomorrow she may not. You must understand the reason for this is that her brain is being destroyed."

That made it clear!

"In spite of this, she may remember you the next day," Dr. Ehrlich added.

I stated my opinion which didn't go over well with the doctor, but made perfect sense to me. If the place where information is stored in the brain is destroyed, I thought, that information is lost and cannot ever be recovered. "There is no way anybody is going to remember anything with a destroyed brain. There is either something holding her memory down, or not bringing it up, but to be able to remember what is gone defies logic."

Right or wrong, that was my immediate premise. Either something, a negative influence of some kind, was interfering with my mother's memory, or the lack of something essential was keeping it from functioning properly. From this point right up until much later, when I began to get very comfortable with her positive changes, we did nothing that contradicted this premise.

That same day, Dr. Ehrlich gave me a talk about Alzheimer's Disease, the neurological significance, the behavioral characteristics, and the general tragic decline that results. Then we addressed the real world and what my plans were for my mother's care. "Who will cook the meals, do laundry, change her, take care of her pills, and take her to the doctors?"

I told her I would.

"You're prepared to take on your mother's personal care?" Dr. Ehrlich asked somewhat incredulously.

"She took care of me when I was young. In return, I'll do the same."

Dr. Ehrlich made no secret of her skepticism. "You don't know what you are taking on."

She was right. I didn't.

Ma's lack of reaction to the preliminary diagnosis was curious at the time. She wasn't out of touch, and she appeared not to believe the doctor's assessment.

So, having heard the diagnosis of "probable Alzheimer's," and armed with my premise and a family history of seeking solutions, I naively set out with every intention of improving my mother's condition.

The Plan

Our family had a lifetime of experiences with doctors and hospitals, most centering around my brother Bob who had spent some part of nearly every year of his life in a hospital. As a boy, the most pressing health problems for Bob were threats of polio, which proved to be unfounded, to rheumatoid heart problems, which were real. Bob survived the ominous prediction of dying from rheumatoid heart problems because my parents acted with decisiveness, seeking out needed experts each time something came up. I have been raised with a family history of choosing to act rather than waiting for something else to happen.

And so, upon hearing my mother's diagnosis, I chose action over inaction.

I have a college background that includes experimental psychology, and from 1962 through 1968 I served in an army reserve medical evacuation hospital. Six years of watching doctors, and being taught something about medical procedures, coupled with an innate curiosity, gave me a perspective that later proved advantageous in coping with my mother's condition.

I had a general understanding of what Alzheimer's Disease was, but my immediate response to the diagnosis was to research the definition of the disease. In the National Institute on Aging bulletin (NIH Publication No. 95-3782, October 1995), "Alzheimer's Disease, Unraveling the Mystery," there was the definition.

The characteristic symptoms acquired a name in the early part of the twentieth century when Alois Alzheimer, a German physician, described the signs of the disease in the brain. Alzheimer had a patient in her fifties who suffered from what seemed to be a mental illness. But when she died in 1906, an autopsy revealed dense deposits, now called neuritic plaques, outside and around the nerve cells in her brain. Inside the cells were twisted strands of fiber, or neurofibrillary tangles. Today, a definite diagnosis of Alzheimer's disease is still only possible when an autopsy reveals these hallmarks of the disease.

I now understood that a definitive Alzheimer's confirmation could only be made by autopsy where the finding of plaques and tangles in the brain could be confirmed. In the meantime, watching my mother lose her mind and seeing her body malfunction and fail was something I would not passively accept. I could not envision putting her in a nursing home where she might languish in a bed or chair, immovable, and wait for the inevitable. Not only that, I could be next and, in addition, I was concerned about my daughter, Anne, and her future offspring. I felt I had no other choice, and it was as much for me as it was for my mother that I formulate and execute a plan of action with the first rule of thumb being to do no harm. This is how I proceeded.

From our dealings in the past, we knew doctors' records on a given patient are often not in one place, as doctors prescribe for their own purposes and retain their own records. It was our experience at the time that some physicians did not know for sure what medications their patients were taking, or had taken in the past. I knew I had to compile my mother's complete medical history for study, both for her physicians who might not be viewing the total picture, and for me.

I collected her medical records from the hospitals where she had been a patient and gathered a reasonably comprehensive listing of her medications. Like most pharmacies, hers was able to print out seven years of her records. We had copies of almost all of her doctors' records that served to back up our memory of her medical history.

Fortunately my mother always carried in her pocketbook a list of her current prescriptions. She never threw out the old lists, as they might come in handy if someone tried to give her a prescription that had already proved ineffective or had produced a negative reaction. We also were aware that some drugs taken years before may have side effects that could crop up months, if not years, later.

Because I think in pictures, I started by envisioning my mother and then listed each ailment or surgery, from head to toe:

- Cerebral Hemorrhage
- Macular Degeneration
- Loss of Sense of Smell
- Stroke
- Broken Clavicle

- Heart Attack
- Pacemaker Installed
- Urinary Tract Infections
- Poor Circulation of Extremities

Our diagrams and records were constantly updated and used as reference throughout her care. The question I asked, of course, was, "What could this information tell us?"

I decided to cut down on the things that might be doing damage, in keeping with my premise that my mother's loss of mental acuity might be a result of negatives in her life. My idea was to get control of as many variables as possible, eliminating the suspected negatives and building on the possible positives. I tried to combine common wisdom with the latest knowledge.

I began substituting "good" foods for "bad." Red meat was limited because it is hard to digest. Whole wheat replaced white bread, since white bread is nutritionally deficient and raises sugar levels dramatically and if sugar has anything to do with her bouts of hyperactivity, we didn't need it. White potatoes had little of the food value we needed; we switched to sweet potatoes. Antioxidants were important to us, so vegetables, colorful vegetables, fit the bill. My mother had always eaten them, and now she ate more of them. The less cooked vegetables were, the more food value they had. Raw would have been the best, but al dente was the rule, so her vegetables were cooked just enough so she would eat them. Since she already had fruit practically every day, I increased the amount and variety.

Chewing food thoroughly was an adage Ma conscientiously honored. When she ate, my mother chewed and chewed. I'd finish eating and be half finished with the dishes by the time she was done with a meal. I had read that chewing food thoroughly aids digestion, so I was happy this practice was already in place.

Preservatives or chemicals in foods were avoided by not eating anything processed: no canned vegetables, no canned fruit, very little frozen. There were a few exceptions. Looking back, I doubt this extreme was necessary, but I had decided to be thorough, so everything was suspect. If I had any reason to think it was bad, that is how it got classified, and thus avoided, most of the time.

Life would have been easier with a microwave, but true to my "good-bad theory," I never bought a microwave, as I thought they destroy antioxidants in food faster than any other cooking method.

The water coming into our house was treated with over ten chemicals to "purify" it. Chlorine alone, at some level, is toxic, and I had no idea how the cumulative effect of chemicals we were exposed to might affect my mother, so in my effort to purge the negatives, even if only suspect, I did away with drinking city water. We used well water, making the assumption that at least it didn't have any added chemicals.

The contents of the water caused me to think about all the other chemicals we are exposed to over a lifetime. Ma had spent her life in her gardens, and I knew she used a powder to eliminate grubs in her iris, something to reduce black spots on the 40 rose bushes, and something else altogether to kill Japanese beetles. Then there were the lawn treatments, feed, weed killer, and garden pest spray. Thus, I stopped using chemicals of all kinds in the yard because even though she no longer worked in the garden, she still visited it.

The house was another matter. There were chemicals everywhere; under the sink, in the bathroom, in the cellar, in the garage. I stopped using all of them, sprays, deodorizers and cleaners, in her presence. This necessitated a lot of late night cleaning after my mother's bedtime, but it was part of the plan to minimize her exposure to any chemicals that might be a part of the problem.

Our plan gave me control over some variables, removed the anxiety that a lack of focus creates, and renewed my hopes. In spite of the grim predictions of Alzheimer's Disease specialists, I did not consider hope harmful, and with my optimism restored, my determination was strengthened and renewed.

THE DARK MONTHS

A few short months after the "probable Alzheimer's" diagnosis, my mother had regressed from scrutinizing the Sunday paper to reading only the headlines. She was not remembering what she read, and would unknowingly reread the same newspaper multiple times. By June she was "reading" the pages sideways and upside down.

Another major change that had gradually occurred in my mother was she had become more passive. The once scrappy lady, who had no problem pointedly voicing her opinion on matters, had become increasingly docile. Just using the word docile and Ma in the same sentence seems an absurdity, but it was a fact she was simply not herself.

Ma was no longer driving, and surprisingly expressed no desire to do so. I knew this behavior saved us one battle which adult children often have with an aging parent, but that was of little consolation to me at the time.

She had also become incontinent. This issue was compounded in the beginning by recurring urinary tract infections. The UTIs were caused by incontinence and her inactivity, which was due to difficulty walking. She had no desire whatsoever to move. The discomfort of the UTIs made her irritable. In the past, my mother was perfectly capable of showing some irritability, and I was used to and perfectly comfortable with it. It was part of who she had always been, and though I had heard others comment about how she sometimes snapped, these moments didn't disturb me in the least. It was part of her personality and I was usually amused by her zeal. But now she would occasionally flare up for no reason, and it wasn't the flaring that bothered me as much as the unreasonableness of it. My mother had always let reason be her guide, and it was this lack of basic logic that disturbed me more than anything. When she was bathed, for example, my mother might get snippy without cause, or perhaps this was her underlying displeasure with loss of privacy and independence. When the UTIs were treated, it became obvious that she was more comfortable, and much kinder.

By July 1996, there was little question of my mother's incompetence.

The woman who had always made decisions with a confident ease could no longer decide what to eat. She had regressed from preparing her own meals to allowing me to do so, with no input from her. She showed no reaction to food in any way and I thought, at first, this was probably connected to her previous loss of sense of smell. Looking back, I am sure it was a contributing factor. Since my mother had always had a distinct dislike of cooking, I would sometimes amuse myself with the thought that she was outsmarting me to avoid kitchen duty. At the time, anything incongruous entertained me as fatigue set in, and I may have chosen feeling amused to avoid feeling overwhelmed. Was this my way of avoiding my feelings about my mother's demise? Perhaps. I suppose suppression of emotion was a comfortable place for me, but at the time I felt I had too much to do to waste time with mental whining.

Only a few months before, her lawyer thought she was fine; now she had lost recognition of time and place.

She had difficulty dressing, was unable to recognize family members, needed assistance walking, suffered loss of appetite, had hallucinations and was mildly, intermittently, combative.

By late July her Alzheimer's symptoms progressed further still. She wouldn't, or couldn't, sleep. She was in what I called an Alzheimer's stupor for hours a day, spending much of that time sitting, staring blankly and mostly unresponsive, on the couch. She did not understand TV, nor could she focus on it. She had stopped gardening and never even looked at her flowers. That upset me more than I can say, probably because the most painful part of this situation for me was the loss of who she had always been, rather than any unpleasantness associated with her daily care.

Another noticeable change concerned my mother's interaction with the family pets. In prior years she had given the appearance of indifference to our animals, but appearances are deceiving, and I knew she cared about them and was constantly amused by them. She had a fondness for our cats and dogs, but for some reason didn't want it known. This was in keeping with our family's inclination toward withholding any appearance of affection. It was apparent that she cared about them as she would ride herd on us kids, making sure we weren't lax in our pet-feeding duties. She would carefully observe the animals and, at the slightest limp, undetected by the rest of us, would promptly usher them to the vet. Other times she would be "caught" patting and ear-scratching the cats and dogs. To put it bluntly, in our household pets weren't exactly spoiled, but they were doted on more than children, my mother's parenting philosophy being essentially hands-off. I think my mother felt offspring were equipped with good sound minds and should mostly teach themselves. But the dogs entertained her, and it was always my understanding that she appreciated and identified with the aloof independence of the cats.

But during her lost months, my mother became indifferent to animals, including our dog Ooste – more evidence that she was drifting away from who she'd always been. Previously she and the dog had an understanding and liked each other. On three occasions, Ooste had shown her connection to my mother by uncharacteristically nestling her head in Ma's lap, apparently sensing something was ailing her. Each time this happened, my mother ended up in the hospital within a day. But at this point, it was not an appearance of indifference I saw in my mother; she simply did not pay any attention to the dog. Ooste would approach her, and my mother would push her away.

We were steadily losing the woman we had always known.

Definitive Alzheimer's Diagnosis

I n the last weeks of the summer during the dark months, Dr. Ehrlich sent us to a neurologist to further verify her earlier diagnosis of probable Alzheimer's. The neurologist did some testing and concluded my mother had Alzheimer's Disease, but our conversation led me to believe he was not an Alzheimer's specialist and, when asked, he acknowledged he wasn't. I explained, perhaps in the same candid way I had inherited from my mother, that we had already received an initial diagnosis of Alzheimer's Disease from her internal medicine doctor, and were there to follow up with a specialist. I insisted that we wanted an Alzheimer's specialist. We got one.

The second neurologist, Dr. Teresa Gomez Isla, who was doing research on Alzheimer's, came on board. In the fall of 1996 she had my mother tested. In the two-hour testing session, which included questions like "Mrs. Pitman, is it day or night?", my mother could not answer one question. She didn't know if it was day or night, or whether she was Mrs. Pitman.

There were agility tests, blood tests, medical tests. Tests, tests, tests, that were spread out over a matter of weeks.

At the same time I was also dealing with conditions at home that had gone from bad to worse. I had to make some decisions on the organization of the household. I decided not to make any major changes. My thought was in order to make things safe, I should do only what was necessary, and as little as possible, in order to maintain familiarity and minimize my mother's anxiety. The only changes I made were small ones, like picking up scatter rugs, in the interest of safety.

My mother had always kept a household of organized stacks of very important material, or so I was told when I chided her to clean up the messes. She read voraciously, cut out articles, and saved them in piles here and there. When she needed something, she could always find it. My decision to retain the familiar surroundings meant leaving piles of newspapers on the couch, the sewing table set up in the living room, as it had been most of my life, and a couple of card tables laden with stacks of "important papers and articles." Boxes of newspaper clippings were in various spots, including the landing on the stairs. The dining room table was covered with flower and gardening information. Under the table were more papers. Though I didn't like it, it was still her house, one of organized clutter – not quite dangerous, but close.

After having given household changes careful thought, imagine my reaction when I came home one day to find a visiting nurse touring the house, making a list of changes for me to carry out. First of all, I was furious that they would be going through the house in my absence, but when they started with their list, I politely showed them the door. Though we did use and came to greatly appreciate the nurses, our first encounters were not as amicable as our last.

And still the tests continued. We were back to the neurologist for more brain scans, and physicians concluded that my mother probably had hydrocephalus and were considering installing a shunt. I suggested they look at the previous brain scans they had in their records. There were two, one by the neurologist who had repaired a cerebral hemorrhage eighteen years earlier and another from two years prior when we were concerned about her loss of sense of smell. However, when they cross-checked the three sets of brain scans, they could find no change. The comparison avoided unnecessary surgery.

They had done all testing available at that time: blood test for thyroid, B-12 deficiency, brain scans, and on and on and on. After this, extensive memory and dexterity testing was done, and the results were interpreted. Thus we ended 1996, months after the initial "probable Azheimer's" diagnosis, with a "definitive" diagnosis of Alzheimer's Disease for my 84-year-old mother.

CHERYL'S CARE

S o this is the journey we traveled, finally reaching the point where our story opened. My mother spent her days virtually uncommunicative and with little or no recognition of her surroundings or her loved ones. Cheryl and I cared for her, doing most everything, as she was unable to perform the basics of self-care. I was trying to execute the only plan that made sense to me, feeding my mother natural, healthy foods, keeping regular doctors' appointments, doing what was necessary to keep UTIs and congestive heart problems at bay, sheltering her from chemicals and toxins that might be unhealthy, and trusting Cheryl to do the same in my absence.

Cheryl was an astute and kind caregiver from the very start. She understood her role well, having worked as an aide in a nursing home. When she first arrived, she saw my mother at her worst – lethargic, her head often on the table. Cheryl was there in case my mother needed something, but her hours of service often involved tediously watching her charge doze on the couch.

Cheryl's first weeks with my mother taught her that firmness was necessary, and early on she told me of the day she had to put her foot down. Cheryl thought that my mother did not take to her for some time as Ma greatly disliked being told what to do. Since my mother was so unsteady on her feet, Cheryl would stand in front, facing her, guiding her down the stairs from the second floor. My mother made it clear that she resented the help. Early on, when Cheryl was guiding her, my mother started to swing her cane in Cheryl's direction, as if saying "Get away from me." In an uncharacteristically firm voice, Cheryl said, "I have to help you. Don't you swing that cane my way again."

Cheryl understood that my mother's need for independence was the cause of her actions, but after her stern words, my mother accepted her presence, her help and, eventually, her friendship.

I paid very careful attention to Cheryl's accounts of my mother's condition and, as weeks passed, she reported on improvements she observed during the hours I was gone.

Corn on the Cob

Concurrent with all of this, something positive had happened.

My mother had a lifelong lunchtime habit of eating an apple, a few crackers, cheese, and a cup of tea. While eating, she read: several newspapers, books on travel, flowers, anything. In her youth, her own mother had told her to chew each mouthful thirty times. My mother did. The leisurely process of lunch took about an hour from start to finish.

Now she was in a daze most of the time. At this point, even though she sat in front of the television regularly, she did not indicate any interest. The TV elicited no response from her; she simply didn't look at it anymore.

In addition, she was losing weight, day in, day out, eating only the equivalent of about one-half of a sandwich per meal. She was incontinent and suffered from colitis and I knew an ear of corn would probably make for repercussions for both of us. The colitis would necessitate frequent changes of her Depends, a less than pleasant routine for caregiver and my mother. But corn was in the fields and Ma loved corn. I'd decided to put up with the inevitable result as a trade-off for the enjoyment she might receive.

I served her an ear of yellow corn and I can only describe her response as rabid. She attacked the corn so voraciously that I decided to step in, thinking she should slow down a bit. Her reaction was extreme. As I reached for the corn, she pulled away and continued to devour it. It was like trying to take steak from an unwilling dog. I was shocked at her reaction, as it was so bizarre and frightening because I had never seen such savagery in her eyes. What a marked difference from the former unhurried pace of her lifelong eating habits.

I had no choice but to allow her to finish, which she did. There wasn't a kernel left on the cob. After she finished the corn, I helped her to her place in the living room. As usual, she went into an Alzheimer's stupor, and awoke about an hour and twenty minutes later to look in the direction of the TV. I asked what she thought and I did a double-take when my mother actually made a comment about the activity on the screen. The blank stare had turned into vague recognition for a fleeting moment. Luck was shining on us. Common sense told us to pay attention to this reaction, and the surprising change.

Though the change might be regarded as trivial, I knew something significant had happened.

AFTER THE CORN

This small response from my mother was the impetus that altered my role in her care. I advanced from manacled caregiver, always looking for something, anything, to do that would help the situation, to caregiver with purposeful direction. Beginning on that very day in July after my mother's simple meal of **yellow** corn (The color turned out to be important), my methods changed, setting a foundation for the logical pursuit of a solution through a specific search for cause and effect.

The next morning I called Dr. Ehrlich, only to be told there probably wasn't any significance associated with the corn. As you may have gathered by now, that was not an answer I was apt to settle for. I persisted with the doctor and was referred to the pharmacy department of the hospital, where I asked what part of the corn might have produced the change. They had no information to offer. Again, this was 1996, and knowledge and accessibility of information about diet and supplements has come a long way during the last fourteen years.

I was convinced that the effect of corn on my mother's behavior was real, and was bent on finding out the nutritional components of corn. I visited our local hospital's dietician, where I received a dietary breakdown of corn. As had become my habit, I consulted with George Elias, our trusted pharmacist, and we both set out to discover what component could be important.

My first suspicion was that simple sugar might be a factor in my mother's change, knowing that some believe sugar can cause increased energy or hyperactivity in children. I soon dismissed the thought because my mother had been consuming numerous foods which contained simple sugar, without any noticeable behavior change.

I researched everything listed in the dietary breakdown. After eliminating the other components in corn, I concluded lysine might be responsible for her change. Lysine is an essential amino acid, and amino acids make up proteins, which are vitally important to our genetic structure. I acknowledge that I am not alone in my theories on such supplements, but at the time, it was a discovery I stumbled upon while relatively disassociated from those pursuing this line of thinking.

George reviewed the pharmaceuticals and supplements which my mother was taking at the time, and after two months of thought and research, he agreed that trying her on a regime of lysine should cause no problem. I was determined to take any action that might help Ma, as long as it would not harm her. Dr. Sullivan consented to its use, and the attending neurologist at MGH was also informed.

Within a few hours of taking the first tablet of lysine, I felt that my mother appeared a bit, a very little bit, more alert. The empty eyes that stared into nowhere seemed to change, very slightly. Replacing the blank stare was a slight increase in eye motion, prompting the thought that she was responding to a stimulus, similar to her response after eating the ear of corn.

After months of darkness bordering on despair, I was almost fearful of the small shaft of light that flickered inside me. I could not shake the thought that things appeared to be looking up. I could only ask myself, "Was it real?"

Urinary Tract Infections, Dehydration, Electrolyte Imbalance

At the same time that I was becoming the tiniest bit hopeful about my mother's mental state, there was a battle going on to balance other factors in Ma's physical condition. There was a recording in my head. Over and over it played: urinary tract infections (UTIs), dehydration, electrolyte imbalance. Which one or what combination was the worst player in the drama of my mother's decline? Was there a causal relationship involved here and, if so, what was it?

Because urinary tract infections were ever present during my mother's dark months, I concluded at the time that they were, at the very least, a part of her dementia problem. Now, as I look back at the course of my mother's struggle with Alzheimer's, I am strongly convinced that these infections were at the very crux of her dementia problems. It was our experience that when her UTIs were raging, so was she. When the UTIs were treated successfully, Ma was more like Ma again.

Do UTIs cause Alzheimer's? I do not know. I do, however, have a strong suspicion that their relationship to dementia is significant. As I made these observations in connection with my mother's problem, I spoke with many people of varied ages who reported feelings of behavioral imbalance when a UTI was present. In normally healthy people, even when the symptoms of burning or urgency to urinate did NOT exist, women, particularly, have described a feeling of anxiety and/or emotional reaction. One usually mild-mannered young woman recalled tearfully demanding to be treated before more serious cases in the ER, a stance completely out of character for her. Another recalled making phone calls and insisting that her medication be processed "THIS INSTANT." Again, an action that was not her usual style, even though she had dealt with typically more serious ailments. And finally, in my extensive contact with Alzheimer's patients during my mother's illness and since her passing, I have found the number of AD patients plagued with chronic UTIs approaches one hundred percent. It is astounding.

During those times before my mother had Alzheimer's and when she occasionally had a UTI, she was often miserable, grouchy, impatient, distracted and sometimes aggressive. So, I wondered, could more dramatic behavioral aberrations, like yelling, hallucinations, night terrors, etc., be what an elderly, more physically compromised person experienced with a UTI and, more specifically, an untreated and/or chronic one?

It is my belief that UTIs play a role in Alzheimer's Disease by acting on proteins and altering their structure and function in some way. I am convinced that UTIs are at least one of the culprits causing the protein changes in AD patients.

While caring for my mother, I found that doctors, nurses and practically every caregiver, professional or amateur, were aware that UTIs contributed to some of the behavior of the dementia patient. Though they all knew of this relationship, for some reason they didn't attribute it to causing dementia, but merely thought of it as a common companion.

The significance of these infections was further reinforced when I visited nursing homes and day care centers where the ever-present UTI problem was often mentioned by the staff members, especially when I brought up the yeast and urine smells permeating the air. I asked why something wasn't done about this problem and the answer was almost universal. The UTIs had become untreatable. I knew that any disease builds a resistance to the cure when it is allowed to build immunity to the drugs that fail time after time to completely cure an infection.

An uncured UTI becomes an incurable UTI.

It was at this point that the severity of untreatable urinary tract infections hit me.

The causes of UTIs are known. Inactivity is associated with the problem. Not drinking enough fluids contributes. Sitting in damp clothing or Depends can spawn these infections. This was the case with my mother.

Previous to her dementia, my mother's occasional UTIs were more easily treated because she was gardening, driving and carrying on a reasonably active life. Not sitting for hours at a time probably helped prevent the return of the infection.

She also had a bladder problem prior to her Alzheimer's diagnosis and had worn Depends on and off for years. Perhaps the occasional damp Depends caused UTIs, which in turn contributed to her development of dementia. As she was failing she did not know enough to change her undergarments and the problem became more serious. From the time we recognized she was not tending to herself when wet, she was changed. We kept her as dry as possible, recognizing that cleanliness came first. While still functional she resisted changing Depends until she was floating; it was a waste of money in her estimation. In spite of this, we did not hesitate to put on new Depends, even if it was a very short time between changes. Changing her did not alone solve the UTIs but did eliminate one of the contributing factors and she clearly seemed to have fewer episodes as a result.

Later, when her strength was waning, and her activities further decreased, the infections increased, requiring immediate treatment. But we discovered that the treatment was frequently unsuccessful, and another UTI would erupt shortly after the treatment for the first. All the while she was becoming more demented. It got so bad that my mother would be screaming and yelling at night, disturbed by hallucinations. This behavior looked like the problems we had seen or heard about from other UTI sufferers. As I gained an appreciation of the seriousness of these infections, and though the doctors didn't seem to hear me, I still became even more convinced than ever that UTIs were a contributing factor to her dementia symptoms.

My first concern was treating this cause of my mother's symptoms in order to see if that would result in positively changing her dementia. If we could permanently cure the infections, would it be possible to do away with these associated symptoms? Would part of the disease disappear? Under the circumstances, if we got a small change, I felt it would be a big improvement and at least a step in the right direction.

We came to this predicament of recurrent UTIs while the doctors were waiting for her to show symptoms or complain about pain before taking any action. Because of her demented state, she was unable to communicate any reason for her behavior. I don't know how many doctors said something to the effect of, "Well she isn't complaining about discomfort."

When she was in full-blown Alzheimer's, I finally said to one, "Ask her her name."

"She can't tell me her name."

"And you expect her to report about a UTI?"

Though we saw the return of her infections, we did not immediately recognize the predictability with which they returned; it was almost immediately after they had been treated. This led me to believe they were not being fully cured in the first place. I noticed that not one of the doctors had rechecked her after treating her to see if they had cured the UTI. They had assumed all was well.

The important thing here is that she be rechecked to see if the UTI had, in fact, been cured.

When my mother became a patient of Dr. Joseph Sullivan, we made an agreement that she would be checked after each UTI treatment, even if she was showing no outward symptoms of an infection. He followed through, and after treating for her next UTI, he took a urine sample to see if she was cured. She wasn't. We needed to be more vigilant in keeping an eye out for these infections. When one was discovered (usually the smell of the urine was the tip-off) she was treated immediately. Then she was rechecked, and treated again if a UTI was still present. Using this plan, we quickly eliminated the problem.

Remember that this was fourteen years ago and, since then, the treatment of UTIs has, of course, improved. However, I am not convinced that rechecking to see if the infection has returned is consistently done today.

In the meantime, however, I wondered about what else we could do to keep the infections away. Could cranberry juice, the old fashioned cure, be the answer? I decided my mother could not drink enough cranberry juice to keep the infections at bay. She always drank cranberry juice and, in spite of that, had developed the infections. George Elias, our pharmacist, came to the rescue again. I asked him if they made a cranberry extract that would do the trick. His answer was yes, a cranberry supplement is available. It was definitely worth a try, but he made no guarantees that it would be effective in preventing my mother's infections. My question was, "Could she take it safely in conjunction with her daily meds?" Again, yes. Cranberry extract was then added to her regimen.

After Dr. Sullivan's successful treatment and follow-up, and by keeping my mother dry, hydrated and "cranberried" up, we got the result we sought. She never had another UTI – not one. She was more agreeable, less distressed, happier, and some of the symptoms of her dementia were gone. What a relief! We seemed to have one problem under control.

I was convinced that the difference in our outcome as compared to others was because of the diligence with which we pursued the problem.

My mother never drank enough fluids and I had learned that, without ample amounts, the urinary tract never gets flushed out sufficiently to prevent bacteria from building up, which had undoubtedly been a contributing factor in causing her infections. We also came to recognize that dehydration alone produced its own problems. The bouts with dehydration that my mother endured gave me the opportunity to observe that behavioral symptoms resulting from dehydration are not unlike those associated with UTIs, except they can become far more serious more quickly. Thus we had identified two antecedents and, I think, contributing causes to my mother's Alzheimer's Disease: wet outside and dry inside.

We could take steps toward solving both aspects of those problems by getting her to drink sufficient fluids.

Things were complicated in my mother's case because of her congestive heart condition. She was taking Lasix, which eliminated the excess fluid in her body and thus caused her to urinate much more frequently than normal. The more she urinated, the greater her chances of dehydration and the increased likelihood of a UTI because she would be wet. This was a delicate balancing act.

Another complication with dehydration is that it can cause an imbalance in the patient's electrolytes. My mother lost potassium, an electrolyte, as a result of the loss of fluids and dehydration. We combatted the low potassium with Klor Kon, a doctor-prescribed, powdered potassium supplement that we mixed in her favorite tonic water. Bananas and more bananas were the other potassium addition to her diet. Such an electrolyte imbalance, for example, too much or too little potassium, can also cause symptoms of dementia and can even cause death. My memory of Dr. Kevorkian made this point more real. I noted that the infamous doctor's method of euthanizing patients was to administer large amounts of potassium chloride in order to end their lives. I could not underestimate the importance of a healthy balance of electrolytes in my mother.

I knew there were lots of other electrolytes to be considered and hoped her new diet was addressing those needs as well. I asked myself if problems with other electrolytes could be part of our problem. That was up to Dr. Sullivan to monitor with his blood tests. His advice was followed, always and unfailingly.

These three problems: UTIs, dehydration and elect-rolyte imbalance, were inseparable. My mother's urinary tract infections underlay her agitation, hallucinations and aggression. They were associated with dehydration and electrolyte imbalance. They caused memory interference and rage, and they affected the protein balance in the body. This was and is my understanding and gave me many reasons to think we might be able to reverse her dementia, or at least some part of it. I never forgot to pay special attention to this troika of diseases because it is my opinion that without their proper treatment, our story would be just like so many others: heartache, dementia ineffectively treated with useless drugs, decay, and death. If this had been our course, I would be emotionally plagued with feelings of unconscionable guilt for not being able to help my mother.

LYSINE

As the doctors, Cheryl, and I continued with my mother's care, we prioritized keeping infections and dehydration in check, and electrolytes balanced. Though I had not mentioned the lysine to Cheryl after the corn on the cob incident and the research that ensued, I remained consistent in adding it to my mother's daily pills.

A few weeks later, when I returned from work, Cheryl commented to me, "Your mother seems different today."

"What do you mean?" I asked.

Cheryl indicated that my mother's eyes seemed more responsive.

I said nothing.

The next day just before Cheryl left for the afternoon, she remarked, "Your mother seems brighter today. The vagueness is not the same as it has been."

Again, I did not respond.

On the third day, the jig was up. Cheryl, who is characteristically a calm and unexcitable person, grew impatient with me. "You're not listening to me." She raised her voice slightly. "There is a change going on here."

At that point I admitted that I, too, was observing the same change in my mother, and told her about the lysine. She could hardly contain her excitement.

As the days passed my mother's eye reaction to her surroundings continued to improve. It appeared that she was returning somewhat, but to hope for too much seemed foolish. I muted my rising optimism and continued with the lysine and a vigilant eye.

MA'S SOFTER SIDE

In the days ahead we seemed to be winning the battle against UTIs, dehydration, and electrolyte imbalance. We were consistent in following our plan of keeping her dry, encouraging liquids, offering her healthy foods, and giving her lysine and cranberry along with her daily medications. My mother had more frequent and longer periods of alertness and, though there was by no means an overnight miracle, her progress was steady and without regression. I almost dared to believe her improvement would continue.

Though she was sometimes cantankerous, the late hours of hallucinations and chaos were but a nightmarish memory. I would have been more worried if she wasn't reasonably grouchy, because she was historically not a warm and fuzzy person. She was intelligent and talented, but also opinionated and frank. And yet...

The mother I remembered so well showed her kindness in sharing what she loved – her flowers. A woman and her husband, both well into their eighties and later in their nineties, drove from Connecticut yearly to view my mother's garden. She gave them and many others the gift of her flowers, separating rhizomes, digging up bulbs, extracting phlox, so they could enjoy her flowers in their own gardens. Each year she gave away hundreds, perhaps as many as a thousand, iris rhizomes.

Though when she was her old self she had little patience with people she deemed lacking in common sense, there were times when I noted her kindness toward people who were less equipped intellectually. There was one such girl who worked at my parents' manufacturing business. She performed her duties to the best of her ability, but her skills were less than expected. Nevertheless, my mother was adamant about keeping this girl in our employ, and she often went out of her way to treat the young woman kindly.

My mother also had a soft spot for animals and accepted and appreciated their quirks. Peanut and Beagle, a duo of beagle dogs, were my parents' boating dogs back when my mother was the first mate and pilot of the boat, and my father, the captain and navigator. The dogs ran the deck, and it was lucky they could swim, as the waves, often as high as eight or ten feet, would occasionally throw them into the water. My mother took tender delight in their hijinks, but she took their rescue seriously also. She was always concerned and, as pilot, would maneuver the boat alongside the pet overboard, supervising as my father wielded a large, long-poled net to retrieve him. The dogs would go right back on the deck for their next swim, and my mother would make sure Dad fetched them from the water again.

Her appreciation also extended to Puffy the cat, who would stand on the deck of the fourteen-foot boat until she was close enough to land, at which time she would jump in and swim to shore. Puffy's maneuver produced admiration from my mother, as would the cat's trips to the jetty, where she'd jump into the surf to catch fish.

Teddy, our collie dog, liked to go flying. My mother and we kids stayed at the Cape house, and Dad flew the sea plane in after his work day. My mother valued Teddy's announcement of my father's arrival, as his barking began long before we could hear or see the plane approaching.

During her illness Ma's latent tenderness began to manifest itself once again.

Cheryl related other incidents that might seem out of character for my mother. One involved the daily weighing. My mother did not enjoy the chore of mounting the scale on a daily basis, but it was important in keeping an eye on the fluid retention involved with her heart condition. She would consistently resist the routine. Cheryl, who witnessed these morning skirmishes, reminded me that even after our "discussions," as I bent over the scale to record her weight, my mother would routinely plant a kiss on my forehead.

Ma was a complex personality. She was refined, yet would swear and state her opinion bluntly and in no uncertain terms. She would suffer fools poorly, yet was open to and enjoyed conversation with everyone. Was there a heart beneath the cool exterior? Yes. Could her demeanor entertain? Yes. Could it also rattle your teeth? Definitely!

So some occasional crabbiness accompanied by periods of alert response from my soon-to-be 85-year-old mother seemed like paydirt to me.

Nursing Homes, Day Care, AD Meetings

Though my mother was having lucid moments and I was encouraged by her progress, I was aware that it could get to the point where I couldn't take care of her. I had no intentions of putting her in a nursing home, but I needed a backup plan in case something happened to me.

Investigating different options, I started by visiting nursing homes because several people had advised me that she belonged in one. Later I explored day care facilities, thinking she might benefit from contact with people outside our home. I looked into, and became a regular at, Alzheimer's meetings in New England.

As I traveled from one nursing home to another, I became increasingly depressed by what I saw. Upon leaving, I felt I would be hard pressed to force myself to revisit them. If the feeling of hopelessness was too much for me, how could I think of subjecting my mother to such a place? I realized that, because I worked for myself, I had options that other caregivers did not. I am aware of the improvements facilities have made in the care of Alzheimer's patients since my visit 14 years ago. Even with these changes, however, they still would not be my choice for my elderly mother.

The last nursing home I visited had an Alzheimer's unit. It was easy to get in, but quite another thing to get out. The door locked behind me as I entered and, in a very short time, I had seen enough. Not only was there no staff member to greet me, there was no one nearby to let me out, so I wandered down a long, deserted hallway hoping to find a nurse. Finally, I approached a nurses' station.

The woman behind the counter looked up from her paperwork and asked, "Mr. Lopez, what are you up to?"

I assured her I was not an Alzheimer's patient and, specifically, not Mr. Lopez.

She was unconvinced, and continued to refer to me as Mr. Lopez.

Unsure of how serious a problem I actually had and a bit curious as to how far this would go, I somehow convinced her to get the supervisor. Unfortunately, as the summoned supervisor approached from another long corridor, she also greeted me from a distance. "Mr. Lopez, what are you doing?"

I waited until she came closer, and explained that I was there researching the place for my mother's possible care, and she did, thankfully, realize I was not a patient. We had a nice chat, and I was glad that it looked like I was not going to be assigned a bed. Obviously Mr. Lopez didn't know who he was, and neither did they.

When my escape was finally facilitated by the supervisor, it was amazing how fresh the air outside smelled to one "Mr. Lopez." Though I was 57 years old at the time, I evidently bore a decent likeness to an AD patient. Maybe I "belonged" there, but it was certainly no place for my mother.

Following up on the idea that it might be good for my mother to get out and see other people, I went to day care facilities that specialized in caring for Alzheimer's patients. The local one had no windows except in the entryway. They were also greatly understaffed, and I left feeling an even greater sense of despair.

My impressions of all the facilities I viewed were similar. The staff in such places was kind, caring, hard-working and well-meaning. They were also over-worked, and stretched too thin for the tasks they were assigned. In spite of that I could not deny what I saw as the futile outlook toward their charges' fate, and it was more than I could take. To try anything beyond the accepted practice seemed a sacrilege, creating false hope. To me hope was never false. On top of that, their jovial demeanor under the circumstances made me uncomfortable.

My observation of the patients was even more disheartening. I viewed human beings who displayed little interaction with one another or their environment. Fear, agitation and discomfort were evident in some as they sat, in wet Depends, smelling of urine, while others seemed overmedicated, unable to hold their heads up. It was never a pretty sight to my eyes. All I could think was, "What a terrible thing to happen!" These visits did nothing to improve my opinion toward this type of care.

Later, after my mother showed reasonable improvement, I attended a meeting at one of the first Alzheimer's centers in the United States. I wanted to see what they would think about what was happening with us. I was careful not to make any wild claims, just observations that could be backed up by our medical or Visiting Nurses Association records. I explained the changes in my mother. The chairing doctor was dismissive, making it clear that he didn't think any good could come from our method of caring for an Alzheimer's patient. He ended by asking, "What are you trying to do, make her live longer?"

My response: "Can you tell me when she's going to die?" Without waiting for his answer, I commented, "If you can tell me, I won't feed her that day."

The family caregivers attending seemed to appreciate the comment, though I'm sure its significance was lost on the doctor. This was confirmed when he went on to explain that Alzheimer's patients can live with declining mental and physical health for an average of eight years, exactly the situation I was trying to prevent.

All of these visits bolstered my resolve to care for my mother at home, and I looked forward to fine-tuning the steps we had taken thus far.

FINE TUNING

Throughout the days that followed I continued with the lysine supplements, and I carefully observed my mother. I noticed that her increase in cognition persisted in the mornings, but decreased by noontime. Some could argue that it was the consistent care she was receiving, which I had little doubt was true, but I was convinced that the lysine was also having a positive effect. After checking with her physicians and pharmacist, I began giving her lysine at noon with her lunch in addition to the morning dose. After a very short time, her alertness extended longer into the afternoon hours.

My mother's behavior had improved significantly at this point. Even the visiting nurses were commenting on the changes in her awareness and ability to communicate. When they came to take her vital signs or draw blood to have her Coumadin levels checked, she showed an increasing participation in the process. "Don't pinch me with that thing," when they put the blood pressure cuff on too tightly. "Use the other arm," she might say, when it was time for them to take blood. These were signs of the person I knew. I was tired, but greatly encouraged, probably excited, if only I'd had the time to realize it.

She was somewhat "with us" most of the day, but as nighttime came, if I hadn't fed her corn with supper, she began to disappear. Was it logical to increase the dosage of lysine by adding another tablet? Off to the doctor and pharmacist again. There was consent, so my mother got lysine at supper time as well, and showed the same improvement at night as in the morning and afternoon. She was now with us all day and, as her periods of acuity grew longer, the degree of alertness improved right along with it.

The reaction to corn was also apparent in two friends' families. The mother-in-law of my neighbor had recently been diagnosed with Alzheimer's. It was Thanksgiving and the matriarch sat at the table and was given an ear of corn. She uncharacteristically devoured it without stopping. There was another woman in similar circumstances, who detested corn. In a conversation with her husband, I somewhat indelicately suggested, "She doesn't know corn from a tree, so feed her some and see what happens." She devoured the first small ear, and did the same with the second. Who knew what this meant? Their behavior seemed significant to me.

I found, after a time, that my mother's degree of alertness in response to corn seemed to level off. It took me a while to suspect that our change from yellow corn to white corn could be the reason. When I went back to yellow corn, we once again got a positive result. I also noticed that corn on the cob was preferred to corn off the cob. My brother had pointed out that chewing is known to increase circulation of blood to the brain, so I left it on the cob, the way my mother preferred it anyway.

My mother loved fish – to catch them and to eat them, especially bluefish. I couldn't stand the smell, so I substituted other types of fish. There had been con-siderable discussion of healthy Omega 3 oil in fish, salmon being one high in Omegas, and she loved it. Of course, since that time the benefits of Omega oils have become common knowledge, but it wasn't then. I began to serve salmon two, sometimes three, times a week because it was supposed to be good for the heart and circulation. What harm could it do?

BREAKTHROUGH

After a few more weeks of continuing the routine, my mother began putting on her own coat, and had started to look at the newspapers, though she was mainly reading only the headlines.

By fall she had progressed to completely washing and dressing herself once again. She took a renewed interest in her gardens and admired and rearranged the flowers I had cut from them and placed around the house. Though still incontinent, she no longer slipped into a stupor at any point during the day, and was sleeping without the persistent insomnia that had previously plagued her at night.

To say I was thrilled with the reemergence of parts of my mother's old self is an understatement. The positive changes strengthened my vigilance and I was determined that if we could get this much progress, then we could also get more.

Marked improvement was clearly evident in her increased awareness and mild displeasure that she expressed during routine trips to the doctor's office.

My mother had an ironic sense of humor that her doctor was not attuned to. He recognized her as a demented old lady only. Though he was always respectful, his understanding of my mother's condition was limited by the brevity of the visit and he was unaware of her rather dramatic changes from one appointment to the next. Nor did he expect any improvement in an Alzheimer's patient.

One time he greeted her. "And how are you, Mrs. Pitman?" He went on to speak to me instead of her while he checked her heart, pulse, and her legs. This was fine when she didn't know what was going on, but things had changed. I knew something was galling her, but could not pinpoint it. Outside the building, she declared, "I don't like how that doctor is talking to me." He had hardly said a word directly to her.

During her next doctor's visit, my mother's disdain for his demeanor grew evident, but only to me. Aware as I was of her sly and sometimes offbeat sense of humor, I suspected she might handle his lack of speaking directly to her in some unusual way.

"Mrs. Pitman, how are you?"

"I'm pregnant," she deadpanned.

Luckily I was sitting behind the doctor, so he wasn't privy to my attempt to suppress laughter, or cover the tears rolling down my cheeks. Part of my response was a result of just thinking this comment was funny. Remember I was raised with the same off-the-grid humor. The other part was an uncharacteristic giddiness at seeing the old Ma once again.

"Mrs. Pitman, do you know where you are?"

"Of course. In your office."

"Do you know who you are with?"

"My son Bradford." (The full name. I guess I was in trouble.)

"Who is the president?"

"That SOB Clinton." She did not approve of his escapade with Ms. Lewinski.

This went on, with my mother firing back answers as quickly as the questions came.

Fifteen or twenty minutes later, the exam and questions were over and the doctor left the room.

"Ma, are you going to let him in on your little pregnancy joke?"

"No. Let him figure it out on his own." She could have cared less what he thought.

I realized that the doctor had to ask the same questions of my mother each visit in order to consistently observe her ability to answer, but I still believe to this day he really had no idea she was putting him on.

THE BETTER TIMES

O nly a few months had passed since my mother's behavior and condition had turned a corner, and she was clearly making steady progress. We kept to our routine day to day, and my mother became more and more alert.

She had started looking at the entire newspaper, and I wasn't sure how much of it she was absorbing yet, but that crept into the picture. One day she commented on a land transfer that concerned my real estate business, and it was then that I realized she was reading and remembering the news.

I was the chief cook, and one advantage to my mother's prior loss of sense of smell was that she ate and appeared to like anything I served her. Though her olfactory ability was compromised, she had the memory of a sense of smell and would comment now and then on how delicious the food was. Encouraged, I started cooking with a bit more imagination. I made spaghetti. My mother's previous idea of spaghetti was canned pasta, which she ate every ten years or so. I now used a prepared sauce as the base of everything I did with tomato-spaghetti sauce because I was still trying to control the variables in an effort to observe what seemed to work, and also because we both liked it. I continued cooking with olive oil because of the supposed benefits to cholesterol levels. Into the oil went lots of chopped onions, garlic, red and green peppers, even though I usually did not feed her things that were hard to digest. This was something she didn't eat very often and

I had no idea if she would eat it now or even whether her stomach would withstand the richness of the mixture.

When I planned and prepared meals for my mother, I never forgot that she was an artist. She had graduated from Rhode Island School of Design, and she sculpted, painted, and created bountiful gardens. She always had flowers in the house, large bouquets of them and, just as often, vases with a single bloom. Depending on the season, it might be a vase with a lone purple iris, a single red rose or a brilliant yellow daffodil. She liked the simplicity of one flower, the better to appreciate its uniqueness. As an artist, color was important to her, and I used it to entice her appetite, especially during the times she had little desire to eat. I also thought that with a diminished sense of smell she might rely more heavily on the appearance of food for allure. I won't say that every plate I served looked like a masterpiece, but I did my best to aim for a humble, colorful work of edible art.

The first time I served spaghetti, I fed her a fairly large meal, trying to encourage her to eat more, but expecting to throw away a good portion of it. She cleaned her plate. She went in and sat in front of the television, and went to sleep for over an hour.

Later that evening, she was holding the newspaper in front of her while TV's Wheel of Fortune was heard in the background. At one point my brother, Bob, was attempting to solve the show's puzzle. My mother suddenly lowered the newspaper, squinted over the top of it, gave the answer to the puzzle, and resumed reading.

It was the corn effect all over again. Since it was the second time I had experienced this type of reaction, it didn't look like pure chance to me. I also knew what to do. I went to the dietician at the hospital again and got the dietary breakdown of tomatoes. Lycopene was the con-centrated antioxidant in processed tomatoes and I thought it could be another beneficial food.

After checking with the medical professionals, on a Wednesday at noontime I gave my mother a soft gel of lycopene, adhering to my guiding premise of trying only what wouldn't harm, and might help. I came back to the house about two o'clock as Cheryl was leaving.

As soon as Cheryl left, Ma looked at me and asked, "Is Hilda's birthday June 23rd?" Hilda was our neighbor of over fifty years.

I said yes. Persisting with the topic, I asked, "When is Bob's birthday?"

"April," she replied.

Me: April what?

She: The fifth.

Me: How about Kendra's? (My sister)

She: Halloween.

Me: How about mine?

She: How the hell do I know?

She'd had enough of this foolish game.

Some might say that this exchange would not be surprising because it involves long-term memory, which is often better in Alzheimer's patients than short-term memory. But recalling that she had no memory at all a few months prior, I considered the conversation impressive.

We were giving my mother her supplements and serving her foods that they were derived from. To our mainstay of yellow corn, we then added spaghetti sauce on a regular basis. I mixed it into several dishes, including chicken, American Chop Suey and meatloaf.

Though my mother wasn't yet completely her old self, we now had the return of a functional person. Could she improve further still?

Time passed with steady uphill progress in her mental health and, in just over a year from her original Alzheimer's diagnosis, the Visiting Nurses notified me that because she was so improved they would no longer be coming.

Spring became summer, and previous summers on the Cape had instilled a love for scallops in my mother. Cape scallops were tiny, sweet, and $28 a pound. Had she known that, she would never have eaten them, but I was pleased that she would recognize them as Cape scallops and appreciate them as her favorite. I was varying the corn and spaghetti, as I had become more confident that things were going in the right direction, so I tossed in an occasional meal of scallops to break up the routine.

The right direction was signaled by the fact that she was coming up with more answers on Wheel of Fortune and Jeopardy. I still didn't know the extent of what she remembered until something cropped up, and these two TV shows were a consistent indicator of her improving mental functioning. Though she wasn't as adept at either of the challenges presented in these shows as before, I was often on the losing end of the competition.

The summer flew by and more progress became apparent as we moved into fall. She was reading the newspapers and commenting on a wide variety of articles. She moved around the house as if it were hers. It truly was, once again.

PAYING ATTENTION

With the pressure off I had time to review what we had done, and to think about what worked and what didn't. If there was one element in caring for my mother that I came to realize was of ultimate importance, it was paying attention. To me, paying attention consisted of three parts: careful, vigilant **observation**; analysis of the information, which included recognizing the likely **reasons** for her behavior; and **acting** on the conclusions drawn from this process. This is not new theory. The hard part is being consistent. However, I believed that if I applied determined effort in each of the three elements, my chances of yielding some success increased. Successes might be small ones along the way, but in our case I considered the end result a substantial success. I would preach to myself over and over the steps in paying attention, simply put: **Observe, Reason, Act**.

It had been my experience that improvements resulted when these steps were followed, and that a missed step in the process had negative, sometimes disastrous, results. I include medical professionals, care-givers, and myself as participants in both successes and failures in paying attention.

We were fortunate enough to have my mother's caregiver, Cheryl, in this story because her powers of observation were impeccable. She carefully reported to me, thus giving me another valuable set of eyes and ears, supplementing my ability to pay attention. My brother Bob, Dr. Sullivan, and George Elias, our pharmacist, all contributed to different aspects of this process in our quest to help my mother get well. It was a small team, but a successful one. I developed the habit of making a list of observations before each doctor's visit. My hope was that such detailed communication with the doctor would give him a complete picture, and increase his chances of drawing the right conclusions.

As an example of how "Paying Attention" didn't work if all steps were not applied, I can go back to the very beginning. I did see signs of Ma's oncoming dementia, the cutting board incident being one of them. At the time, I executed step one **(observation)**. Where I failed was in allowing confusion to prevail, and in not putting the warning signs together **(reason)** and in doing nothing **(action)**. I performed one out of three steps. I can excuse myself here, saying that it was too early to jump to conclusions at that point, and perhaps it was. I could ask, what could I have done way back then? Take Ma to the doctor and explain that she had wrecked my childhood gift? I use this as an example of the necessity of performing all three steps, but it also serves to show the complexities that enter into the process.

I observed instances of the breakdown in the "paying attention" paradigm in the medical community as well. One example is in the way UTIs were often dealt with. I thought doctors and nurses could not help but observe the consistent presence of UTIs in Alzheimer's patients. But I did not, at the time, see any attempts to further examine the link between the condition and AD. And what about reaction to what was observed? Yes, there was an attempt to cure the UTI, but in our experience, lack of consistent rechecking to see if the infection was indeed cured was the breakdown in step three, **acting** with determination in order to reach a permanent resolution of the problem.

I do recognize that there are so many areas of concern for medical professionals to deal with that the odds of missing a step are increased exponentially. I, however, was caring for one patient, and could press for cooperation in seeing that all three steps were consistently carried out. This gave me comfort, as did the attitude of at least some of the medical professionals who indicated they appreciated that we were on the same team and thought my efforts worthwhile.

There were times when I knew I had executed all three steps. My mother's reaction to corn on the cob was one incident where paying attention was beneficial. Step one: I observed her rabid response to the corn. I didn't dismiss it. There was a change in the light in her eyes when she looked in the direction of the TV, which did not go unobserved. Step two: I put these incidents together and I researched corn. There was some reason she attacked it ferociously at a time when she had minimal interest in food. There was some need in her body that made her react. After researching I concluded it might be lysine. Step three: I gave her a tablet of lysine. The three steps of "Paying Attention" were completed. It is worth mentioning here that, after this, I began again at step one in carefully observing her reaction to the supplement, drawing conclusions about dosage, and carrying out adjustments. I just didn't want to miss anything.

There were other examples where paying attention elicited positive results: the x-ray comparisons of her brain,

Dr. Sullivan's recognition of the overmedication for her congestive heart condition, and on and on. The point is made how all three steps were inherent in effectively dealing with my mother's condition. Clearly, my experiences have proven time and again that "paying attention" and carrying out all three steps is the most valuable of any caregiving tool I can think of.

During the writing of this book, I fell prey to a breakdown in the steps of paying attention. I was going through a period of fatigue and not feeling as mentally sharp as usual. Did I observe? Yes. Did I make connections and react? Not immediately. After a visit to the doctor, I learned I had a UTI! Of all people, I was acutely aware of this malady and its symptoms, but I failed to "pay attention" in my own case. A humbling experience, and one I vowed not to repeat.

Is it possible to be infallible in "paying attention?" Probably not. However, it enhances the chances of prudently solving problems. Is it possible to be consistent in "paying attention?" In my mind, yes.

I know being consistent didn't make us perfect, but it gave us the best chance we had, and certainly improved the odds of getting a better result. The success with my mother that resulted was worth the determination and effort, and the spirit of hope that prevailed changed the everyday life of all involved.

It is my firm belief that if caregivers and medical professionals "pay attention" in this way, a loved one who has been diagnosed with Alzheimer's Disease might still be able to "come to the party."

PINEAPPLE

It was the pre-Christmas season, and a neighbor appeared one night with an offering of a fresh pineapple. I had just fed my mother her evening meal, a sizeable helping of spaghetti with meat sauce. I cut up the pineapple and placed a bowl of it on the table next to her on the couch. She claimed she was full and couldn't eat it. "Just leave it then," I said.

I went to clean up the kitchen a bit and when I returned about three minutes later, the bowl was empty. The speed in which the good-sized portion of pineapple was dispatched did not go unnoticed by me. For her to eat something when her appetite had already been satisfied and after she had refused the fruit was not her usual habit. She fell asleep and awoke an hour later.

Her answers to Alex Trebek's challenges that night were on the mark. I even recall some of the categories of that night's game. She knew which countries certain rivers of the world passed through. She was a demon in the category of Travel, as well as Art, and came up with artists' names and where they had painted certain works. When I questioned her further on a particular response, she expanded on the "obvious" differences in the style of two Impressionists.

I had always noted as a child that my mother's answers, though often terse, were quicker and more on target than those of her contemporaries. She would fire off swift, succinct responses on a variety of subjects. You don't see that as often in the elderly, and the habit that had amazed me in my youth not only amazed me once again, it tickled the hell out of me.

The night of the pineapple was another particularly bright moment for my mother that I paid attention to. We know well that our body is equipped to fight disease and that innumerable responses occur within us in attempts to right the wrongs imposed upon our good health. Even to the scientist, the systems that kick in to aid recovery must seem miraculous. Why then do we not pay close attention when the body's appetite talks to us? We see it, but ignore it. At this point I dismissed nothing I observed in my mother's behavior as unimportant.

I didn't have to puzzle too long over the incident. I researched pineapple, and found bromelaine, an enzyme believed to have positive effects for numerous health issues. I checked with the professionals, was assured it was safe for my mother, and added it to her daily intake.

I proceeded with confidence because it was the third time I had made such an observation. It was the same song played over again, first with corn, then with processed tomato, and now with pineapple. The mystery of the first and second experiences was somewhat diminished with the third. It seemed obvious and simple to me at this point. My reaction was more like "There it is again." When it happened this time, I can't say it was expected, but it was not at all beyond my belief, and I was not afraid to take unbridled pleasure from it as one does from the replay of an old sweet song.

HER OLD SELF

M y mother's journey for the past year had been a long one. She had been diagnosed with Alzheimer's Disease, suffered a period of the darkest times of her life in a state of vacancy and unresponsiveness, been hospitalized and placed briefly in a geriatric neuro-psych ward, and then had steadily become more alert, more active, and more her old sharp-minded self. By the end of her 85th year, she was back.

There were many moments that transpired in the next two years of her life that made me smile and reminded me how good it was to have her with us once more.

One such moment was her last appointment with her AD neurologist. It was a telling visit and a short one. He greeted her in the same manner as he had on her initial visit. Unlike their first meeting though, she carried on a normal conversation with him.

He went through a thirty-question verbal test. She scored eight points higher than her test six months prior, at a time when she had only begun improving, and would continue to progress even more as weeks passed. There is no doubt in my mind now that she would have achieved a perfect score in the months that followed if we had bothered to return to him for another visit.

I asked if such a marked improvement was typical.

He seemed to not know how to respond. I suspect because he had no precedent to support an answer. He wrote out a prescription for Aricept, though I would not use it for her and the visit was over. Time to move on.

As we exited, and once out of earshot, my mother turned to me and commented, "We drove all this way for that?"

At a later date we also made a return visit to my mother's former internist. Because of the distance involved during the height of my mother's problems, we had changed to a local doctor. Now, though, I thought she would like to see the change in my mother. After the visit I asked Dr. Ehrlich for a letter describing any change she saw in my mother's condition over the last twenty months. In reference to the earlier visit, her letter stated "At that time she had fairly severe symptoms of AD..." And after this visit, the doctor wrote, "I have seen Mrs. Pitman on June 10th, 1998. At that time she was markedly improved, alert, able to concentrate, able to tell a joke, answering questions well, previously she had been unable to answer questions. Good short term memory and logic." This is a simple but striking report of two visits to this doctor.

Another moment which highlighted my mother's marked improvement and which showed me she was indeed back and ready to take charge once again concerned her daily pill routine. One day, about six months after her condition improved noticeably, I took stock of the supplements and medication she was taking, and because she was doing so well, I made the decision to eliminate one of the two folic acid tablets from her daily intake. I brought my mother her pills and, as usual, she placed them on the table, moving them around, obviously grouping them according to some system of her own, the order of which I never bothered to ask. She had spent a lifetime classifying all manner of things, and I knew she had her reasons. Suddenly she looked up from her work, and commented, "Where's that other little white pill?" as though she had caught me being less than conscientious about my job as caregiver.

"I'd like a list of my medications again, so I can keep track of my own pills!"

I was amused by her comments because it showed how astute her power of observation was compared to just months ago, and because I remembered well when she was not only disinterested in which pill was which, but would lick them up off the table, a practice I was glad she didn't remember.

Another habit that surfaced during this period when my mother was again her old self wasn't reported to me until after her death. Though she was doing well by now, I still wanted Cheryl there when I was out of the house working. She was present for company, if my mother needed something, or in case of emergency. By this time they had become good friends, and though Cheryl was no youngster, my mother had taken to calling her "kid."

"Would you like a lollipop, kid?" It was the first of many times she would offer, and Cheryl was surprised to see her unearth a stash of literally hundreds of lollipops. Of course high-sugar foods were not on my most recommended list, and Cheryl couldn't imagine how she had amassed, and obviously now remembered the whereabouts of, such a collection. Feeling fairly certain that I was unaware of the hidden treasure, Cheryl accepted it as one of their little secrets, and she related that it wasn't unusual for my mother to read the paper or watch the news with a lollipop stick protruding from her mouth. I thought I knew where Ma's candy supply was, but evidently I had been outfoxed again.

Cheryl reminded me of another of my mother's quirks, which she resumed after her absence from normalcy. My mother would "decorate" the downstairs bathroom mirror. It was a standard-sized medicine cabinet mirror, and she would tape clippings of jokes onto its surface. The result was only about a two by four inch rectangle of mirror left in the center, barely enough for a view of one's eyes. She got a kick out of guests visiting the bathroom and reacting to all this. Cheryl particularly liked this habit because it was a perfect example of the way my mother could embrace clutter, coupled with her unique sense of humor.

Even though I knew her improved behavior was real, I still found myself pleasantly surprised by the normal little words or actions she showed me on a daily basis. I suppose we appreciate what was once lost more when it returns, and seeing my mother thrive again put a smile on my face every day.

Ma's Return in Retrospect

In retrospect, I realize that my mother's cognitive return probably first revealed itself as she began to recognize who she was once again, a short time before she recognized any of us. Why do I think this? I recall minute examples of her changing behavior. She began to straighten her clothes, or sweep the hair out of her face again. She would fidget when the couch wasn't just the way she wanted it, or straighten a picture on the wall. All these actions had been absent for too long.

People ask me what the exact period of time was when my mother's subtle changes were in evidence, but the precise time of her return is harder to pinpoint than her disappearance. It was an ever-changing series of events which just crept up on me. I can only say that her improvement started in the last quarter of her sabbatical from life as she knew it, and my mother's recovery was incremental as time passed, discoveries were made, and changes were implemented. She had lost her mind gradually; she regained it gradually, until the good times began to outshine the bad, and life became typical for our household with a person who was, bit by bit, my mother once again.

Co Q 10

B y spring of 1998 my mother, now eighty-six years of age, had been enjoying good mental health for about a year. I could see nothing that indicated that she wasn't her old self, though her heart, of course, was still a serious problem, making it hard for her to get up and down the stairs. My ninety-five-year-old friend had an opinion on that. He suggested we look into the coenzyme Co Q 10. Before my mother slipped into her mental abyss, she had only taken a multi-vitamin along with her prescribed medications, and I had never taken a supplement of any kind in my entire life. I was, and still am, not totally convinced that there is magic in supplements. In my mind, if it works, good; if not, forget it.

So with my usual skepticism, I looked into Co Q 10. It is an antioxidant that is reported to be responsible for human body energy and to support heart muscle strength. I thought it was worth a try. The pharmacist and doctor were consulted and again it was agreed that it would not be unreasonable to give my mother Co Q 10. It was added to her pills.

My mother's process for climbing the stairs to her bedroom was to take a few steps, and then stop and rest. I was accustomed to hearing the clump of a step or two, then silence. Her steps, then silence.

After about five months I was considering dis-continuing the use of the Co Q 10 because I hadn't seen any evidence that it was helping.

One night, however, as I busied myself in the kitchen, I realized I had not heard any of my mother's typical step-climbing sounds. When I investigated, I found her halfway up the stairs! Evidently the progress had gradually occurred without me realizing and, all of a sudden, there it was.

She continued to get Co Q 10. It was the last thing to be added and was the only change made from some months before. Had it helped her? Though I felt the Co Q 10 was a contributing factor, I also knew her overall improvement in health was instrumental as well. In any case, I was satisfied with the effects of Co Q 10 and the improvement in her stair-climbing ability.

Business as Usual

L ife in my mother's home now proceeded along smoothly. She was interested again in the activities of the ski club and the iris club. She received visitors, some couples that she and my father had known for years, neighbors, and other acquaintances. She had always enjoyed lively conversations with a variety of people, and now that these occasions were again part of her life she presided with her usual spunk. She manned the front door at Halloween, distributing candy to the trick-or-treaters that year. "Come in here, and let me get a good look at those costumes."

My mother's improved health gave me the gift of time, and that year I worked to catch up with my real estate work; I subdivided some plots of land, and cut out a road for a local company. My ski equipment business was running along, and I kept busy filling orders for the upcoming season. Later, during some leisure time while my brother was at the house, I began skiing again.

The household had returned to normalcy; even the gardens flourished.

One afternoon I walked into the house and my mother was sitting in her usual chair playing with her hearing aids. That shouldn't seem odd, but the truth was, I had not seen those hearing aids in over a year and a half.

They had gone missing during the time when things were of the worst for my mother. I was too busy to keep track of their whereabouts, and though I tried asking her if she knew where they were, it was futile because she had no understanding of my questions at that time. I had gone on a mission to find the missing hearing aids, systematically searching in every nook and cranny of the house, first in all likely areas, and then in odd places – everywhere I could think of. I went through every drawer in her room, hunted through her dress and coat pockets, and emptied and examined the contents of her pocketbooks. I searched inside her shoes, and even took the mattress off the bed. You name it. I turned the house upside down.

I had been planning to get her new hearing aids and, as I think about it now, I am remiss that it took me so long to do so. My focus had been elsewhere, and she could hear without them, but not as well as with, of course. So when she was her old self again, and I entered the room and saw her matter-of-factly changing the batteries of the hearing aids, I was surprised and glad that we wouldn't have to go to the inconvenience and expense of replacing them.

In her returned state of alertness, she apparently had remembered that she had hearing aids and retrieved them. Amazing how the mind works. She dismissed my questions about where they had been hiding with a look that said, "Don't waste my time," and I didn't press it. To this day, I have no idea where she'd hidden those blasted hearing aids. Maybe with the lollipops?

Shortly after the resurfacing of the hearing aids, my mother had a routine doctor's appointment. I only recently learned from Cheryl the details of the trip home. It was certainly much different, and obviously more fun, for my mother anyway, than the visits we had made one to two years before. The appointment was some 20 miles from home, and since Cheryl was the one who assisted my mother when nature called in public places, we decided that she would make the trip with us.

The appointment was uneventful, and afterward my mother suggested we stop for lunch at a restaurant.

Cheryl has called me a Type A personality, and though she sometimes mentions my attributes, waiting patiently is not usually on the list. After ordering, my mother decided it was time to visit the ladies' room, so off they went. They were gone forever. Our food arrived and I waited, and waited, and waited. "What in God's name could they be doing in there?" I thought. Since I was seated within earshot of the ladies' room, I could detect sporadic bursts of laughter from behind the closed door, so I felt whatever the holdup was couldn't be serious. I began to pick at my now-tepid meal.

After what seemed an eternity, the two of them returned to the table. I had finished my meal, and was feeling more than ready to hit the road. They sat, giggling like a couple of schoolgirls, and began nibbling at their lunches. Like my mother, Cheryl is an famously slow eater, so my patience was sorely tested as I waited for them to eat at their own leisurely pace. Each time they made eye contact, the laughter would begin anew, and that extended the meal even longer.

Cheryl's account has now filled in the blanks of what occurred in the restroom, as I was slightly peeved at the time and did not inquire. Evidently, once inside the stall, it took some maneuvering to roll down the layers of clothing:

Depends, regular underwear, long underwear, pants. It was taking a bit of time, but Cheryl was never one to rush my mother. In the midst of it all, somehow the toilet paper roll popped off the holder, hit the floor, and rolled. And rolled. Out of the stall and several stalls down.

As Cheryl tells it, my mother started first. The more she laughed, the more Cheryl laughed, and moving the whole operation along swiftly during the hysterics wasn't an option. They finally put her and everything else back together again, and returned to a cold lunch and a bewildered escort.

I suppose I have included these incidents for a few reasons. Not only do they show how normal and full my mother's life had become but, for me, it underscored the contrast. The humorless, vacuous husk of a woman who stared into nothingness months before was nowhere in that restaurant. Instead was my mother, whole and complete, in nearly every aspect.

TULIPS

My mother customarily had 1,500 to 2,000 tulips blooming at any one time in her garden, but there was a lady in Norfolk, MA who had 30,000 tulips all around her house. The word was that she even dug them up each year and replanted them annually, so this was far more than the four or five thousand my mother would have in her stores in order to keep 1,500 flowering in her garden simultaneously.

Now that she was feeling good for her eighty-six years, she remembered the Norfolk tulips, and expressed a desire to see the spectacular display again. She had to do very little convincing to get my brother Bob to take her on a road trip to seek out the tulip house. My brother had always continued his visits with my mother, through good periods and bad, and now that she was fairly healthy, they enjoyed each other's company again.

The weekend arrived and they were off to see the flowers. Bob is usually pretty good with directions, so up Route 115 they went, with my brother taking a right here, and a left there.

When they neared their destination, my mother said, "Bob, you just passed the road we're supposed to take."

"No, it's the next one, Ma."

"It's back there," she insisted.

Around and around they went, both verbally and throughout the neighborhoods.

Finally, my mother lost her cool and told him where to go — and then where to drive the car — in the direction she felt the flowers bloomed.

My brother is not easy to convince, so he persisted in his way, with my mother getting madder and madder by the second.

As she told me later, "The damn fool had no idea where he was going. It was exactly where I had told him."

She had been right all along, and I suspect this was my brother's first firm reintroduction to his mother of yore. Long gone was the sheepish lady who looked for reassurance that she was heading in the direction of the bathroom in her own home. Ma was in the driver's seat, figuratively, once again.

CALL HOME

By November of 1998, not only had my mother been walking up the stairs by herself with relative ease for some time, other improvements were obvious and long-time friends could see no difference in the person they always knew, rather than the lost Alzheimer's patient. She was doing extraordinarily well.

Because it seemed like the time was right, I decided to travel to Europe for a week, leaving my mother in the trustworthy hands of Cheryl. Everyone was comfortable with this arrangement, particularly my mother, as their relationship was by now a close one.

During my trip I called home from a sidewalk phone in London to check on my mother.

"Where are you?" she asked.

"You know where I am."

"You sound like you're standing in the middle of the damn road!"

"I practically am!" I responded. "The double-decker buses are whizzing by me less than a few feet away."

"Where are you going now?" was her next question.

"I'm heading to the ski show." That satisfied her. She knew that the show was one of the reasons I had gone on the trip. There were more questions. How big is the

show?   Where   were   the   exhibitors   from?   Were   any
Olympians going to be there?

After that I described the Bentley that was parked
across the road. My mother loved such automobiles, which
in her estimation were steps above a mere car. Her father
had owned the best, including a Stanley Steamer, and he
had taught her to drive at age thirteen. I supposed it was
from him that she inherited her appreciation of a good
automobile.

After more chitchat she closed with, "I had to send
Cheryl home. She put up quite a fuss, but there was no
need of her staying here to make me dinner, when she has
a family of her own to feed."

"There was no one there to make your meal?" I
asked.

"I made my own supper. She'll be back later on
tonight."

I was surprised at first, but then realized that Cheryl
might have had some authority when my mother was in a
weakened state, but now that she was healthy, few were
up to the task of changing my mother's mind once it was
made up. I was assured from the rest of our conversation
that all was well at home.

Unbeknown to me, things were even better than I
thought.

When I returned from Europe, Cheryl and my mother
picked me up at the bus station, and it was obvious that my
absence had done no one any harm. They were doing that
same giggling I remembered only too well from our lunch

weeks before, and I learned that there were nights when they stayed up late, talking and laughing like kids at a sleepover. Later, Cheryl told me about some of these conversations, and I learned about incidents and information concerning my mother's mother and other relatives that she had never shared with me.

When Cheryl later recapped the week for me, she made it clear that although she prepared meals, did laundry, and helped at bedtime and with medications, my mother was the one in charge.

Cheryl described the first night, mentioning that, as she settled into the guest bed, my mother appeared in her doorway in her nightie, all five feet of her, "sweet-faced and eyes bright blue." "Kid, do you have enough pillows in there?" Cheryl said there was no doubt about who was the lady of the house and, at that moment and others, ironically and enjoyably, Cheryl felt as though she were the one being taken care of.

The next morning, Cheryl languished in bed a little late, until she heard, "Are you ever going to get up?" from the next room. That was the last morning she slept in during her stay.

From the reports I got, the rest of the week was a bit of a vacation for both of them. Meals together, the nightly news, Lawrence Welk reruns, and lengthy chats before bed.

"However, I was beside myself," Cheryl said, "when late one afternoon, your mother informed me that she wanted me to go home and make dinner for my own family.

I knew that I was responsible for staying with her for the entire week, but she led me to the door and pushed me out!"

"I didn't want to leave. You had employed me to stay with your mother day and night, and it wasn't in me to neglect that commitment, but Maude was simply not a force to be ignored. I sat in my car for a very long time, agonizing over what to do. Finally, I went home."

I could see she was fearful that I would be disturbed that she had allowed my mother to overpower her better judgment.

It pleased the hell out of me and I responded quickly, "Cheryl, you had no choice." No one understood better than I that even the most resolute were no match for my mother when she was wearing her game face.

THE BACK HALL

The back hallway of our house became the setting where we inadvertently observed my mother's good health, or lack of it. The typical route for friends and family would be to enter the back door of the house, and if no one was at the table, cross through the kitchen, and proceed down the back hall into the living room.

Bernie, my friend from junior high school days and later the accountant for my business, would always take this route.

I remember one such entrance, during my mother's worst times, when Bernie walked into the kitchen, just as my mother's head dropped into her plate. When she righted herself, her glasses were covered with food, prompting a little cleanup on my part. Though she and Bernie had known each other for many years, she had no recognition of him that day.

Months later, after my mother had improved, Bernie entered through that same back hallway. She was in the living room, and as he and I headed downstairs to the cellar, he called hello to her.

Without hesitation, she said, "Bernie, get in here."

The conversation that followed was as if there had been no interruption in her memory. He was a bit surprised.

Previously, her head was in her plate; now, she playfully bantered with my friend just like the old days.

Another such incident involved Dale, another former classmate of mine. In fact, our families had known each other for years; my father and his were classmates, and our grandfathers were also acquainted. It was during her bad months and, in spite of all their history, I knew my mother wouldn't recognize Dale when he came up from South Carolina for a visit. I warned him ahead of time, and she didn't know him when he came through the hallway.

A year later, after my mother's return from the dreamlike state she had been in, Dale came back for another visit and, because of her marked improvement, I was eager to see her reaction to him.

Through the hallway and into the living room he came.

She looked up. "Whitey, what are you doing up here? Come in! Oh, who's this?" Dale's southern belle, "Bobbi," was right behind him. "Sit down. So what brings you here?"

As the conversation moved along, Dale told my mother they were in town to get headstones for his parents' graves.

"You know, the elder Mrs. Beggs just died," said my mother. She had owned the local gravestone enterprise.

"No, Ma," I interjected. "It was the daughter who passed away."

"The hell it was," she said.

"You're mistaken. It was the daughter, Ms. Beggs." I felt she was confusing the two generations.

"Get the newspapers," she said.

I got the paper to end it all, certain I was right. Well, I wasn't.

It was obvious that she remembered what was going on day to day, as Mrs. Beggs' death had appeared in the papers prior to Dale's visit. This was one of many instances that illustrated how acute her short-term memory was. She was just as accurate as she had always been, and I realized she was working with the same sharp mind I had known all my life. I knew I'd better be at the top of my game from then on.

We sat and talked for an hour or so. The discussion went to how Dale liked living in South Carolina. Though my mother had known, before her dazed period, where Dale and Bobbi resided, it was heartwarming to see that she knew all of this information once again. It seemed as though the intervening bad months didn't exist for her. There wasn't a beat missed in the conversation.

Later, in June of my mother's eighty-seventh year, approximately one month before her death, I entered the house through the back hallway to hear my mother whistling a song from *South Pacific*. I stopped, shocked to realize that I hadn't heard that whistle in many years. It immediately brought me back. In the car, in the house, in the yard, Ma whistled. And that day, the melody that drifted into the back hall was as clear as it had always been. It was an experience similar to the return of her singing voice, but signified to me another layer of her reconnecting with her old healthy, happy behavior.

Though I can hear that perfectly pitched whistling to this day, at that moment in 1999, as viewed from the back hall, my mother looked and sounded darned good.

SATISFACTION

M y mother's return to good mental health had a ripple effect on my life. Friends were more regular visitors at the house, as I had the time, energy and inclination to socialize once more. I continued making the trek to New Hampshire to ski regularly, and had no worry about what was occurring at home in my absence, as Bob was there with my mother and they were enjoying themselves. Though I am not a jump-and-shout kind of person, I reveled in my uplifted mood and felt as close to calm as I get.

I was reminded of the comfort I took in my mother's good mental state when I looked at a picture I took on the trip to Europe in 1998. I had snapped the photo at St. Margaret's Church near Westminster Abbey, in London, while I waited with the crowd of people who had gathered in anticipation of the arrival of the Queen Mum. She emerged from the car, tastefully attired in hat, coat, gloves, and even a low-heeled shoe, a surprise to me because I knew she had broken her hip ten months prior. There were attendants at her beck and call, and a golf cart, painted with her racing colors, was stationed nearby. I knew the cart was there to save her the trek around The Field of Remembrance where she would pay her respects to those who had sacrificed their lives during the world wars.

I was amused to watch her graciously ignore the attendants' attempts to escort her to the cart. She was having none of it, and avoided their efforts to coax her into it. She went about greeting people and then proceeded to walk around the crosses which marked the fallen, for over an hour, bad hip or no bad hip.

At the time I thought, "Now there's a lady who has the same spirit as my mother." She was going to do exactly what she was going to do in spite of the well-intentioned plans of others, just as my mother was not to be deterred when she shoved Cheryl out the door back home. The similarity of the two mums made me smile then, and whenever I look at the picture of the scene, I smile just as broadly.

JULY 14, 1999

It was July 14, 1999, and my mother was delighted to receive an invitation from a Hummel Club friend who was having the members to her house for their annual get-together. Any excuse to go out would be enough for her, but she particularly liked parties. The friend lived in an old home on Cape Cod, and my mother was looking forward to seeing the house, and even more excited about reconnecting with the old gang again since she hadn't seen this group of friends since before her dark times.

Her heart was failing by this time and she fatigued more easily but, motivated by the promise of a party, she gave herself a shower, got dressed, and came down for breakfast. Bob took her to the hairdresser, and off they went to the Cape, my mother looking pretty spiffy all dressed up.

The party didn't disappoint. The club members sat outside, talking and eating, with my mother gabbing and enjoying herself immensely.

She and Bob arrived home late in the evening and he headed back to his apartment in the Boston area and, though exhausted, Ma wanted to talk. She was eager to tell me who was there, what was said, and all about the variety of food presented. She raved about the T-bone steak, and I remember thinking it was probably a nice change from what I, her personal chef, had been serving of late.

She even complained about the bathroom, something she had always done in the past. The light switch for the bath in the antique house had an unusual hidden location, and she commented on the "damn switch" still being hard to reach. To me, the fact that she remembered where it was located was one of those pleasant reassurances that her mind was as good as we thought.

I listened for a few hours, hesitant to cut short a day she had so obviously enjoyed, but as her report ran down, she was finally willing to go to bed.

I got up the next morning and went downstairs to make breakfast. It was unusually quiet upstairs, as my mother normally would have been heading to the bathroom by then. I went up to investigate, and found my mother, in her nightgown, slouched against her night stand on the floor next to her bed. Her heart had stopped when she was either getting into or out of bed.

One consoling thought is that the last day of my mother's life was full of some of her favorite activities, and a far cry from not knowing who she was. She had survived a cerebral hemorrhage, a stroke, her heart stopping, macular degeneration, a diagnosis of Alzheimer's, and ended a life well lived with an acute mind, a last admiring look at the purple Asiatic lilies that bloomed in her garden, and an invigorating day with friends.

I would have liked to have had her around longer.

To this day I am comforted by the thought that I could not have done more to help my mother, and by the fact that during the final years of her life she was cogent and fulfilled. The dark months were a time period lost, but not missed, and I count as an additional gift the fact that once my mother returned to her self and to us, Ma had no memory of when she had no memory.

It had been three years and a world away from the day in July of 1996 when a simple meal of corn on the cob pointed us in the right direction.

Perspective is a mighty force, and I now value and enjoy life with more intensity, and any present difficulties pale in comparison to those times.

THE LAST STEP

Eleven years have passed since my mother's last day, giving me plenty of time to reflect upon what had transpired over a lifetime, and specifically upon what occurred during those years when I was my mother's caregiver. I have spent more than a decade reviewing the written documentation I kept during her care. I have filled file cabinets and my computer's hard drive with information on dementia, Alzheimer's, medication use, and nutrition. I have attended endless lectures and meetings, have spoken at local clubs, given a series of talks at community centers, visited hospitals and nursing homes, and have been in close contact with children of Alzheimer's patients and the patients themselves. All this resulted in a need to pass on our experience, as I believe my mother's story is an uplifting and inspiring one, worthy of being told.

I am, however, an unlikely author. During my high school days I was near the bottom of my class, and with good reason. Unknown to my teachers and others, I could not read. I had some sight words in my arsenal, and my method of preparing for tests was to skim down information in a textbook, recognize a few words in each paragraph, and fill in the blanks from what I had gleaned of the subject in practical situations. It was a less than successful approach, but one that got me a diploma. I knew I had a logical mind and could grasp the essence of a problem, but I also knew something was wrong. I diagnosed my own dyslexia as it was many years before such knowledge and resources had made their way into school systems. After high school, I attended a junior college, where I took a reading course. Something clicked and I learned to read. After that I made up for lost time by reading everything I could get my hands on and continue the practice to this day.

In my case, aggressive reading did not translate as well as I would have liked into improving my ability to write, making a book a more difficult option for me than for most. But the desire to disseminate the good I saw in our experience was worth trying to overcome my writing problems. Though I had the thoughts, putting them on a page so that others would understand my meaning was a craft I needed some help with, so I found someone to work with me on that. The book is a collaboration. The content is mine, the voice is mine; the organization and writing are mine and that of my co-writer, Nancy Driscoll.

Why have I chosen to write this book, when writing is not my natural form of communication? First, my mother's story is, I think, unique, in that though she was diagnosed with Alzheimer's Disease and visited oblivion for a year, she regained her sharp mind, and lived to enjoy it for two more fulfilling years. If there is another story out there that chronicles such a success, I have not found it. Every book I have seen about Alzheimer's or dementia tells the tale of dire predictions and steady decline. But I witnessed and participated in the opposite, and I want all to know it occurred.

I have a need to tell what I have learned. I was educated by the experience of my mother's care, and I have developed strong beliefs about dementia, which is sometimes labeled Alzheimer's, and the care and prevailing attitude towards it. One of these attitudes that

I question is why the focus on the negative? Is it wise to notice only the lapses in dementia patients and accept those as an indication of their destined decline, while dismissing their moments of brightness? My experience taught me to focus on the alert moments, try to decipher what might have triggered them, and work from there. Isn't this just as legitimate a scientific response to the problem as the opposite approach? Why not work for a reversal, rather than accept the notion of sure decline? Each approach takes a similar amount of energy, but ours brings with it positive elements for caregivers, win or lose. The bottom line is it worked for my mother.

Many books have been written on this subject, but rarely from a son's perspective. I hope that my rendering might give voice to a gender and generation substantially affected by their loved ones' dementia. At 70, I have the need that comes with age to continue to be useful, and carrying out this project satisfies that need for me.

A less than altruistic reason for wanting this story told is that I carry my mother's genes, as do my daughter and my grandchildren. I have a vested interest in the care and treatment of Alzheimer's patients and in the future research of the disease. I would be remiss if I did not tell everyone and anyone who will listen, my mother's story.

Acknowledgements

Dr. Joseph B. Sullivan and our pharmacist, George Elias, helped facilitate my mother's unique medical outcome.

The many Boston doctors and other medical professionals did the legwork that kept my mother alive and healthy.

My co-writer, Nancy Driscoll, took my scribbles and translated them into understandable English.

My brother, Bob Pitman, was there to look after, worry about, and enrich our mother's life with trips to restaurants, flower gardens and club meetings.

Cheryl Neal, a one-of-a-kind caregiver, accepted my intensity and helped me survive the everyday turmoil.

The Nolans: Jack, Adrienne, Evan and Alysson bolstered my endurance by giving everything from friendship to legal advice, and much in between.

Allana helped make my first newspaper articles readable.

Linda Shepherd edited and refined our story.

Martha Horn, Priscilla Jane Huston, Sam H. Davis, and John Buchanan read and critiqued our early effort.

Friends and acquaintances who sent articles on Alzheimer's Disease, which filled gaps and led me to further research.

Individuals attended my lectures and their participation, questions, and points of view deepened my understanding.

Others followed our path, offering enlightenment and encouragement.

Phil and Karen Marak who provided wordsmithing, feedback, word processing and layout.

My daughter Anne and husband Greg, and granddaughters, Sarah and Ella are the reasons for pursuing a solution to my mother's dementia.

My heartfelt thanks to all of you.

Authors

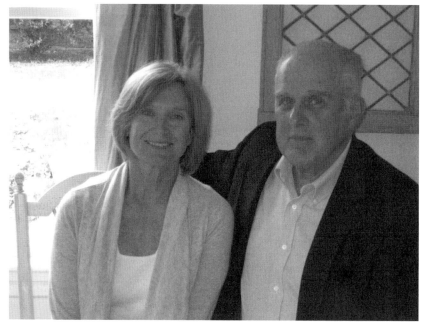

Courtesy Jeanette Caldarone

Brad Pitman has lived in Attleboro, MA his entire life. A businessman and gardener, Brad has dedicated the last 14 years of his life to researching Alzheimer's.

Nancy A. Driscoll is a retired teacher and writer living in Attleboro, MA.   ndriscoll74@comcast.net